Anaphylaxis

Anne K. Ellis

Editor

Anaphylaxis

A Practical Guide

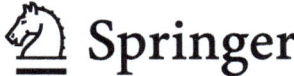 Springer

Editor
Anne K. Ellis
Queen's University
Kingston
ON
Canada

ISBN 978-3-030-43204-1   ISBN 978-3-030-43205-8   (eBook)
https://doi.org/10.1007/978-3-030-43205-8

This Springer imprint is published by the registered company Springer Nature Switzerland AG
The registered company address is: Gewerbestrasse 11, 6330 Cham, Switzerland

Contents

Contributors

Waleed Alqurashi Division of Emergency Medicine, Department of Pediatrics, University of Ottawa, Children's Hospital of Eastern Ontario, Ottawa, ON, Canada

Marcella Aquino Rhode Island Hospital/Hasbro Children's Hospital, Warren Alpert Medical School of Brown University, Providence, RI, USA

Erin Banta NYU Winthrop Hospital, Division of Rheumatology, Allergy & Immunology, Mineola, NY, USA

Anne K. Ellis Queen's University, Kingston, ON, Canada

Stanley Fineman Emory University School of Medicine, Atlanta Allergy & Asthma, Vienna, VA, USA

Shannon French, MD, FRCPC McMaster University, Hamilton, ON, Canada

Catherine Hammond Department of Pediatrics, Allergy/Immunology, University of Tennessee Health Science Center, Memphis, TN, USA

Jay Lieberman Department of Pediatrics, Allergy/Immunology, University of Tennessee Health Science Center, Memphis, TN, USA

Nicole B. Ramsey Department of Pediatrics, Division of Allergy and Immunology, Icahn School of Medicine at Mount Sinai, New York, NY, USA

David R. Stukus Division of Allergy & Immunology, Nationwide Children's Hospital and The Ohio State College of Medicine, Columbus, OH, USA

Julia E. M. Upton Division of Immunology and Allergy, Hospital for Sick Children, Toronto, ON, Canada
Department of Paediatrics, University of Toronto, Toronto, ON, Canada

Julie Wang Department of Pediatrics, Division of Allergy and Immunology, Icahn School of Medicine at Mount Sinai, New York, NY, USA

Tonya Winders Allergy & Asthma Network, Global Allergy & Airways Patient Platform, Vienna, VA, USA

Introduction to Anaphylaxis Essentials

1

Shannon French, Anne K. Ellis

Introduction

Anaphylaxis is a life-threatening severe systemic allergic reaction. It is caused by the rapid release of mast cell mediators into systemic circulation. It is most commonly triggered by foods, insect stings, medications, and latex. It is typically a clinical diagnosis with an acute onset. Anaphylaxis was initially described in medical literature in 1902 during a study which involved immunizing canines with jellyfish toxin. These injections resulted in a systemic allergic reaction in certain animals, rather than protection from their vaccine. This resulted in the term "anaphylaxis," which is derived from the Greek words "ana" (against) and "phylaxis" (protection) [1]. Anaphylaxis requires urgent recognition and treatment. Intramuscular epinephrine is the mainstay of treatment and should be administered as early as possible, with secondary measures to include H1 and H2 antihistamines, corticosteroids, IV fluids, oxygen, and bronchodilators. A period of observation is required following treatment. Atopic individuals are at a higher risk of developing anaphylaxis, such as those with asthma.

Signs and Symptoms

The presentation of anaphylaxis can be extremely variable. Symptoms generally start within 30 minutes of exposure to the triggering allergen, but may occasionally be more delayed. Early symptoms can be mild; however, they may quickly progress to a severe reaction. The signs and symptoms of anaphylaxis typically follow a uniphasic course; however, biphasic reactions do occur. Biphasic reactions have been

S. French
McMaster University, Hamilton, ON, Canada

A. K. Ellis (✉)
Queen's University, Kingston, ON, Canada
e-mail: Anne.Ellis@kingstonhsc.ca

© Springer Nature Switzerland AG 2020
A. K. Ellis (ed.), *Anaphylaxis*, https://doi.org/10.1007/978-3-030-43205-8_1

Table 1.1 Signs and symptoms of anaphylaxis

Cutaneous/subcutaneous/mucosal tissue
Flushing, pruritus, urticaria, swelling, morbilliform rash, pilor erection
Periorbital pruritus, erythema and swelling, conjunctival erythema, tearing
Pruritus and swelling of the lips, tongue, uvula/palate
Pruritus in the external auditory canals
Pruritus of the genitalia, palms, soles
Respiratory
Nose: pruritus, congestion, rhinorrhea, sneezing
Larynx: pruritus and tightness in the throat, dysphonia and hoarseness, dry staccato cough, stridor, dysphagia
Lung: shortness of breath, chest tightness, deep cough, wheezing/bronchospasm Cyanosis
Gastrointestinal
Nausea, cramping abdominal pain, vomiting, diarrhea
Cardiovascular
Chest pain, palpitations, tachycardia, bradycardia, or other dysrhythmia
Feeling faint, altered mental status, hypotension, loss of sphincter control, shock, cardiac arrest
CNS
Aura of impending doom ("angor animi," uneasiness, throbbing headache, dizziness, confusion, tunnel vision; in infants and children, sudden behavioral changes, such as irritability, cessation of play, and clinging to parent)
Other
Metallic taste in the mouth
Dysphagia
Uterine contractions in post-pubertal female patients

Adapted from Ref. [2]

described to occur in approximately 4.6% of all anaphylactic events, based on a recent 2015 systematic review and meta-analysis [2]. Cutaneous findings are the most common symptoms in anaphylaxis, occurring in 80–90% of all episodes [3]. Signs and symptoms of anaphylaxis are listed in Table 1.1.

Diagnostic Criteria

Anaphylaxis is predominately a clinical diagnosis. Criteria for defining anaphylaxis were developed in 2004 by a panel of experts at the National Institutes of Health, which resulted in the publication of the NIAID/Anaphylaxis Network Definition of Anaphylaxis. The determined criteria for anaphylaxis are listed in Table 1.2 [4]. A study by Campbell et al. was done in 2012 to validate the criteria provided by the NIAID meeting. This study provided a sensitivity of 97%, specificity of 83%, negative predictive value of 98%, and positive predictive value of 69% for these criteria [5].

Epidemiology

The incidence and prevalence of anaphylaxis vary worldwide, with differences dependent on a number of variables. Anaphylaxis is likely underreported as well [6]. A 2006 report on anaphylaxis in the USA from the American College of Allergy Asthma and

Table 1.2 Clinical criteria for diagnosing anaphylaxis

1. Acute onset of an illness (minutes to several hours) with involvement of the skin, mucosal tissue, or both (e.g., generalized hives, pruritus or flushing, or swollen lips-tongue-uvula) and at least one of the following:
   (a) Respiratory compromise (e.g., dyspnea, wheeze-bronchospasm, stridor, reduced PEF, or hypoxemia)
   (b) Reduced BP or associated symptoms of end-organ dysfunction (e.g., hypotonia [collapse], syncope, or incontinence)
2. Two or more of the following that occur rapidly after exposure to a likely allergen for that patient (minutes to several hours):
   (a) Involvement of the skin-mucosal tissue (e.g., generalized hives, itch-flush, or swollen lips-tongue-uvula)
   (b) Respiratory compromise (e.g., dyspnea, wheeze-bronchospasm, stridor, reduced PEF, or hypoxemia)
   (c) Reduced BP or associated symptoms of end-organ dysfunction (e.g., hypotonia [collapse], syncope, or incontinence)
   (d) Persistent gastrointestinal symptoms (e.g., crampy abdominal pain or vomiting)
3. Reduced BP after exposure to a known allergen for that patient (minutes to hours):
   (a) Infants and children: low systolic BP (age specific) or greater than 30% decrease in systolic BP

Simons et al. [3]

Immunology (ACAAI) anaphylaxis workgroup quoted a lifetime prevalence between 0.05% and 2% [7]. In the 2006 NAIAD report, the incidence of anaphylaxis was reported to be approximately 10–20/100,000 population per year [8]. However, a 2013 European systematic review on the epidemiology of anaphylaxis reported incidence rates for all-cause anaphylaxis between 1.5 and 7.9 per 100,000 person-years. This review estimated that 0.3% (95% CI 0.1–0.5) of the population experience anaphylaxis at some point over the course of their lives [9]. It has been described in the literature that anaphylaxis is becoming more frequent, with a study by Rudders et al. citing a 58% rise between 2000 and 2009 in the USA [10].

Pathophysiology

Reactions which are described as "anaphylaxis" are classically thought of as being immunoglobulin-E (IgE) mediated, with non-IgE-mediated reactions being dubbed "anaphylactoid." Clinically, these two types of reaction are identical. It has been proposed by the World Allergy Organization (WAO) that the term anaphylactoid be discarded. Instead, the WAO has proposed that anaphylactic reactions be categorized as immunologic and non-immunologic. Immunologic anaphylaxis is typically described as IgE mediated, with non-immunologic anaphylaxis being a result of sudden basophil or mast cell degranulation in the absence of immunoglobulins [11].

The traditional IgE-mediated mechanism of anaphylaxis begins with an antigen binding to an allergen-specific IgE. Antigen-bound IgE in turn binds to the receptor Fc-epsilon-RI on mast cells and/or basophils. This causes these cells to degranulate, releasing a number of inflammatory mediators. These inflammatory mediators include histamine, tryptase, heparin, chymase, cytokines (i.e., tumor necrosis factor,

IL-4, IL-13), prostaglandin D2, leukotriene B4, platelet-activating factor (PAF), and the cysteinyl leukotrienes LTC4, LTD4, and LTE4. Histamine and tryptase are two of the most abundant preformed granule mediators released by mast cells and basophils during episodes of anaphylaxis. Release of these mediators causes the symptoms which are seen in anaphylaxis, such as vasodilation, angioedema, bronchial smooth muscle contraction, urticaria, and pruritus [12, 13].

Differential Diagnosis

The differential diagnosis for anaphylaxis is broad and is age dependent to some degree. Table 1.3 includes a number of entities which can mimic anaphylaxis [2].

Table 1.3 Differential diagnosis of anaphylaxis

Common disorders
Acute generalized urticaria and/or angioedema
Acute asthma
Vasovagal syncope (faint)
Panic attack/acute anxiety attack
Aspiration of a foreign body
Cardiovascular events (myocardial infarction, pulmonary embolus)
Neurologic events (e.g., seizure, cerebrovascular event [stroke])
Shock
Hypovolemic
Cardiogenic
Distributive (e.g., sepsis, spinal cord injury)
Obstructive (e.g., pulmonary embolism, tension pneumothorax, cardiac tamponade)
Excess endogenous histamine
Mastocytosis/clonal mast cell disorders
Basophilic leukemia
Flush syndromes
Perimenopause
Carcinoid syndrome
Autonomic epilepsy
Medullary carcinoma of the thyroid
Postprandial syndromes
Scombroidosis
Anisakiasis
Pollen-food allergy syndrome
Food poisoning
Caustic ingestion (children)
Other nonorganic disease
Vocal cord dysfunction
Hyperventilation
Psychosomatic episode
Other
Nonallergic angioedema (hereditary angioedema, angiotensin-converting enzyme inhibitor-associated angioedema)
Systemic capillary leak syndrome
Red man syndrome (vancomycin)
Pheochromocytoma (paradoxical response)

Investigations

Individuals with suspected anaphylaxis should be referred to an allergist. In a recent review of 573 patients with anaphylaxis seen in the emergency department, only 38% were subsequently seen by an allergist [13]. The diagnosis of anaphylaxis begins with a detailed history. Particular attention should be paid to potential triggers and exposures the patient encountered prior to the event, with foods being the most common cause of anaphylaxis in children and young adults [14]. The timeline of the events leading up to the event is also critical. Typically, anaphylaxis will occur within minutes to hours from the exposure; however, there are exceptions to this. Anaphylaxis to red meat, triggered by IgE antibodies to the carbohydrate galactose-alpha-1,3-galactose (alpha–gal), may often occur 4–6 hours following ingestion [15].

Events occurring prior to the episode should also be addressed, such as exercise [3] or menses [16], which can be the solitary trigger of anaphylaxis. It is also important to review any medications which the patient may have been exposed to in the 24 hours prior to the episode. Medications may indeed be the trigger of anaphylaxis; however, certain medications increase the likelihood of developing an anaphylactic reaction to a separate trigger, such as NSAIDs [14]. Also, patients taking beta-adrenergic blockers may be at a higher risk of severe anaphylaxis or having anaphylactic reactions which are more difficult to treat [17].

Furthermore, there are certain risk factors and health conditions which increase the risk of fatal anaphylaxis. These risk factors vary according to the cause of anaphylaxis. Fatality secondary to food-induced anaphylaxis most commonly occurs in the second and third decades and is also associated with delayed administration of epinephrine [18]. Pulmonary and cardiac disease such as poorly controlled asthma and coronary artery disease increase the risk of fatal anaphylaxis [14, 19]. Mast cell disorders also increase the risk of fatal anaphylaxis [20].

While anaphylaxis is largely a clinical diagnosis, there are certain laboratory investigations which can be helpful when drawn in the acute setting. The utility of serum tryptase has been published in the 2011 NICE Clinical Guideline on Anaphylaxis [21]. Tryptase is produced by degranulation of basophils and mast cells [22]. Tryptase levels rise within minutes of an anaphylactic reaction and peak between 30 and 90 minutes. Their half-life is approximately 2 hours [23]. An elevated tryptase has been associated with anaphylaxis, which generally returns to baseline following resolution of the episode. However, a normal tryptase does not rule out anaphylaxis [24].

Other mediators of anaphylaxis which are currently being studied include histamine, cysteinyl leukotrienes, prostaglandins, and platelet-activating factor. Histamine is mainly stored and produced by mast cells and basophils, but is also produced by monocytes, neutrophils, keratinocytes, T lymphocytes, and enterochromaffin cells [25]. Histamine can cause many of the symptoms of anaphylaxis, including pruritus, cutaneous flushing, airway obstruction, bronchospasm, and hemodynamic changes [26]. Elevation in plasma or urinary histamine is seen in anaphylaxis. However, as with tryptase, normal levels do not exclude anaphylaxis.

The majority of histamine is metabolized to N-methylhistamine and then to N-methylimidazole acetic acid within minutes. Urinary histamine metabolites have also been shown to be elevated following an episode of anaphylaxis [27].

Cysteinyl leukotrienes and their metabolites have also been found to be elevated in the urine during episodes of anaphylaxis [28]. Cysteinyl leukotrienes are made by a number of cells, including mast cells, basophils, and macrophages [29]. There are three main bioactive cysteinyl leukotrienes, which include LTB4, LTC4, and LTD [30].

Prostaglandin D2 is the main cyclooxygenase product released by activated mast cells during anaphylaxis; however, it is not released by activated basophils. Prostaglandin D2 can contribute to the hemodynamic changes seen in anaphylaxis [31]. Elevated urinary prostaglandins have also been associated with anaphylaxis [32].

Lastly, platelet-activating factor (PAF) is a phospholipid-derived mediator which is secreted by several cell types, including mast cells, macrophages, platelets, eosinophils, neutrophils, monocytes, and endothelial cells. It also plays an important role in anaphylaxis and has been found to be elevated in the serum during anaphylactic episodes [33].

Diagnosis

Following the acute setting, once a patient is assessed by an allergist, skin testing and serum-specific IgE testing can be used to determine potential causes of IgE-mediated anaphylactic episodes. Skin prick testing (SPT) is generally the first step and can be done for most foods, venoms, and penicillin. SPT has a negative predictive value of >90% [34]. However, while SPT is quite sensitive (~90%), it has a lower specificity at approximately 50% [35]. A positive SPT is described as 3 mm greater than the negative control [36]. Intradermal testing for food allergy is not recommended due to the risk of anaphylaxis and the high false positive rate [37].

Serum-specific IgE levels are another important diagnostic method used in the assessment of IgE-mediated anaphylaxis. Higher IgE levels correlate with an increased risk of a true allergy; however, higher values do not necessarily mean that a reaction will be more severe. This test is not affected by antihistamines and does not carry a risk of anaphylaxis, which is very rarely seen with SPT [38]. The sensitivity and specificity vary for IgE testing, depending on what allergen is being tested [39]. Skin testing and serum-specific IgEs are often used together in determining the cause of anaphylaxis.

Management

The mainstay of treatment for anaphylaxis in the acute setting is intramuscular epinephrine, at a concentration of 1:1000. This can be repeated every 5–15 minutes as needed, if symptoms persist. If the patient is not responding to intramuscular epinephrine, cautious administration of intravenous (IV) epinephrine is recommended. This should be done in a monitored setting. If IV access is not readily available, intraosseous (IO) access is then recommended. Administration of intramuscular epinephrine should not be delayed, with multiple studies demonstrating an increased risk of a biphasic anaphylactic reaction with delayed use of epinephrine [40, 41].

Oxygen should be administered to any patient with signs or symptoms of cardio-vascular or respiratory compromised and should be considered for all patients with anaphylaxis. The airway should be monitored closely, and intubation should be considered if needed. If there is evidence of circulatory compromise, IV fluid resuscitation should be commenced with normal saline. Inhaled beta-agonists should be considered if there is evidence of bronchospasm. Adjunctive medical therapy may include H1 and/or H2 antihistamines and corticosteroids, but these should not be used prior to or in the place of epinephrine.

It is important to stress that these adjunctive medications are indeed secondary to epinephrine use. Antihistamines in particular are frequently used in the acute management of anaphylaxis and in post resuscitation care. In many episodes of anaphylaxis, antihistamines are given prior to administering epinephrine, which should not be the case. A Cochrane review demonstrated that there is no consistent evidence to support antihistamine use in the acute setting of anaphylaxis [42]. However, antihistamines have been shown to be helpful in the treatment of cutaneous symptoms, such as urticaria and pruritus, and thus it is reasonable to use them once the patient has been treated with epinephrine and stabilized. If antihistamines are used as an adjunct medication, it is preferable to use second-generation, nonsedating H1 antihistamines, which tend to last longer and have a lesser side effect profile. First-generation H1 antihistamines are not generally recommended, as they are associated with more sedation, anti-cholinergic effects, cognitive impairment, and QTC prolongation, compared with second-generation antihistamines. There is no conclusive evidence to support the use of H2 antihistamines in the acute setting of anaphylaxis [43].

Systemic steroids are also frequently used in the treatment of anaphylaxis; however, a Cochrane review demonstrated that their use in the acute setting is not supported by any high-quality evidence [44]. This is logical, given that the onset of action of systemic steroids is several hours. Multiple studies have been done which show potential benefit with steroids in reducing the risk of a biphasic anaphylactic reaction; however, further research is needed [40, 45].

Following resuscitation, an individual should be monitored for 4–8 hours in the emergency department; however, there is significant variability in observation times across various centers [46, 47]. A systematic review on biphasic anaphylactic reactions showed that the mean time between the first and second phases of a reaction was approximately 8 hours [48]. It is therefore reasonable to consider longer observation times in the emergency department. Patients should be counseled regarding the risk of a biphasic reaction and provided with a prescription for an epinephrine auto-injector. Patients should preferably have access to an epinephrine auto-injector promptly upon leaving the emergency department, especially those at risk of a biphasic reaction. Unfortunately, evidence demonstrates that the frequency of epinephrine auto-injector prescribing could be improved. Several studies show that the prescription rates of epinephrine auto-injectors in the emergency setting are between 17%

and 27% [49, 50]. Ideally, all patients should also receive training on how to accurately use an epinephrine auto-injector from a qualified healthcare professional.

If a specific trigger is suspected, this should be avoided until the patient can be assessed by an allergist [51]. A referral to an allergist is an important component of the management of anaphylaxis to allow for follow-up and further investigation, which can help prevent further anaphylactic episodes. Unfortunately, rates of referrals to allergists following treatment of anaphylaxis are not ideal, with several articles quoting rates between 12% and 18% of patients with anaphylaxis [49, 52]. Having an anaphylaxis action plan in the emergency department has been shown to improve referral rates to outpatient allergists, along with improving the rate of prescription of epinephrine auto-injectors [50].

Conclusion

In conclusion, anaphylaxis is a potentially life-threatening allergic condition which can present with multiple symptoms. It can be both immune (IgE) and non-immune mediated. The diagnosis of anaphylaxis is based on clinical assessment; however, there are certain laboratory tests which aid in diagnosis. Anaphylaxis should be treated with intramuscular epinephrine, supportive management, and adjunct medications as needed. The mainstay of management is avoidance of triggers and to carry an epinephrine auto-injector. A prescription for an epinephrine auto-injector should be provided following treatment of anaphylaxis, and training should also be provided regarding its use. Patients should also be assessed and followed by an allergist.

References

1. Fouju G. Fouilles au domaine de Menouville (Seine-et-Oise). Bulletins de la Société d'anthropologie de Paris. 1902;3(1):54–7.
2. Lee S, Bellolio M, Hess E, Erwin P, Murad M, Campbell R. Time of onset and predictors of biphasic anaphylactic reactions: a systematic review and meta-analysis. J Allergy Clin Immunol Pract. 2015;3(3):408–416.e2.
3. Simons F. Anaphylaxis. J Allergy Clin Immunol. 2010;125(2):S161–81. https://www.jacion-line.org/article/S0091-6749(09)02854-1/fulltext.
4. Sampson HA, Munoz-Furlong A, Campbell RL, et al. Second symposium on the definition and management of anaphylaxis. J Allergy Clin Immunol. 2006;117:391e397. IVa.
5. Campbell RL, Hagen JB, Manivannan V, et al. Evaluation of the NIAID food allergy and anaphylaxis network criteria for the diagnosis and management of anaphylaxis in ED patients. J Allergy Clin Immunol. 2012;129:748e755. IIb.
6. Sclar DA, Lieberman PL. Anaphylaxis: underdiagnosed, underreported, and undertreated. Am J Med. 2014;127(1):S1–5. https://doi.org/10.1016/j.amjmed.2013.09.007.
7. Lieberman P, Camargo CA Jr, Bohlke K, et al. Epidemiology of anaphylaxis: findings of the American College of Allergy, Asthma and Immunology Epidemiology of Anaphylaxis Working Group. Ann Allergy Asthma Immunol. 2006;97(5):596–602.
8. Sampson HA, Munoz-Furlong A, Campbell RL, et al. Second symposium on the definition and management of anaphylaxis: summary report—Second National Institute of Allergy and Infectious Disease/Food Allergy and Anaphylaxis Network symposium. J Allergy Clin Immunol. 2006;117(2):391–7.

9. Panesar S, Javad S, de Silva D, Nwaru B, Hickstein L, Muraro A, Roberts G, Worm M, Bilò M, Cardona V, Dubois A, Dunn Galvin A, Eigenmann P, Fernandez-Rivas M, Halken S, Lack G, Niggemann B, Santos A, Vlieg-Boerstra B, Zolkipli Z, Sheikh A. The epidemiology of anaphylaxis in Europe: a systematic review. Allergy. 2013;68(11):1353–61.
10. Rudders SA, Arias SA, Camargo CA Jr. Trends in hospitalizations for food-induced anaphylaxis in US children, 2000–2009. J Allergy Clin Immunol. 2014;134(4):960–2, e3.
11. Johansson S. Revised nomenclature for allergy for global use: report of the Nomenclature Review Committee of the World Allergy Organization, October 2003. J Allergy Clin Immunol. 2004;113(5):832–6.
12. Kemp S, Lockey R. Anaphylaxis: a review of causes and mechanisms. J Allergy Clin Immunol. 2002;110(3):341–8.
13. Campbell RL, Park MA, Kueber MA Jr, et al. Outcomes of allergy/immunology follow-up after an emergency department evaluation for anaphylaxis. J Allergy Clin Immunol Pract. 2015;3:88.
14. Lieberman P, Nicklas R, Randolph C, Oppenheimer J, Bernstein D, Bernstein J, Ellis A, Golden D, Greenberger P, Kemp S, Khan D, Ledford D, Lieberman J, Metcalfe D, Nowak-Wegrzyn A, Sicherer S, Wallace D, Blessing-Moore J, Lang D, Portnoy J, Schuller D, Spector S, Tilles S. Anaphylaxis—a practice parameter update 2015. Ann Allergy Asthma Immunol. 2015;115(5):341–84.
15. Commins S, Satinover S, Hosen J, Mozena J, Borish L, Lewis B, Woodfolk J, Platts-Mills T. Delayed anaphylaxis, angioedema, or urticaria after consumption of red meat in patients with IgE antibodies specific for galactose-α-1,3-galactose. J Allergy Clin Immunol. 2009;123(2):426–433.e2.
16. Bauer C, Kampitak T, Messieh M, Kelly K, Vadas P. Heterogeneity in presentation and treatment of catamenial anaphylaxis. Ann Allergy Asthma Immunol. 2013;111(2):107–11.
17. TenBrook J Jr, Wolf M, Hoffman S, Rosenwasser L, Konstam M, Salem D, Wong J. Should β-blockers be given to patients with heart disease and peanut-induced anaphylaxis? A decision analysis☆. J Allergy Clin Immunol. 2004;113(5):977–82.
18. Turner P, Jerschow E, Umasunthar T, Lin R, Campbell D, Boyle R. Fatal anaphylaxis: mortality rate and risk factors. J Allergy Clin Immunol Pract. 2017;5(5):1169–78.
19. Triggiani M, Patella V, Staiano RI, et al. Allergy and the cardiovascular system. Clin Exp Immunol. 2008;153 Suppl 1:7.
20. Theoharides TC, Valent P, Akin C. Mast cells, mastocytosis, and related disorders. N Engl J Med. 2015;373:163.
21. National Institute for Health and Clinical Excellence. Anaphylaxis: assessment to confirm an anaphylactic episode and the decision to refer after emergency treatment for a suspected anaphylactic episode. NICE clinical guideline 134. London: National Institute for Health and Clinical Excellence; 2011.
22. Jogie-Brahim S, Min HK, Fukuoka Y, et al. Expression of alpha-tryptase and beta-tryptase by human basophils. J Allergy Clin Immunol. 2004;113:1086.
23. Schwartz L. Tryptase, a mediator of human mast cells. J Allergy Clin Immunol. 1990;86(4):594–8.
24. Caughey G. Tryptase genetics and anaphylaxis. J Allergy Clin Immunol. 2006;117(6):1411–4.
25. Salem A, Rozov S, Al-Samadi A, et al. Histamine metabolism and transport are deranged in human keratinocytes in oral lichen planus. Br J Dermatol. 2017;176:1213.
26. White M. The role of histamine in allergic diseases. J Allergy Clin Immunol. 1990;86(4):599–605.
27. Stephan V, Zimmermann A, Kühr J, Urbanek R. Determination of N-methylhistamine in urine as an indicator of histamine release in immediate allergic reactions. J Allergy Clin Immunol. 1990;86:862.
28. Ono E, Taniguchi M, Mita H, Fukutomi Y, Higashi N, Miyazaki E, et al. Increased production of cysteinyl leukotrienes and prostaglandin D2 during human anaphylaxis. Clin Exp Allergy. 2009;39:72–80.
29. Peters-Golden M, Gleason MM, Togias A. Cysteinyl leukotrienes: multifunctional mediators in allergic rhinitis. Clin Exp Allergy. 2006;36:689–703.

30. Austen KF. The cysteinyl leukotrienes: where do they come from? What are they? Where are they going? Nat Immunol. 2008;9:113–5.
31. Butterfield JH, Weiler CR. Prevention of mast cell activation disorder-associated clinical sequelae of excessive prostaglandin D(2) production. Int Arch Allergy Immunol. 2008;147:338.
32. Nassiri M, Eckermann O, Babina M, et al. Serum levels of 9α,11β-PGF2 and cysteinyl leukotrienes are useful biomarkers of anaphylaxis. J Allergy Clin Immunol. 2016;137:312.
33. Vadas P, Perelman B, Liss G. Platelet-activating factor, histamine, and tryptase levels in human anaphylaxis. J Allergy Clin Immunol. 2013;131:144–9.
34. Sicherer SH, Sampson HA. Food allergy. J Allergy Clin Immunol. 2010;125(2 Suppl 2):S116–25.
35. Sampson HA, Albergo R. Comparison of results of skin tests, RAST, and double-blind, placebo-controlled food challenges in children with atopic dermatitis. J Allergy Clin Immunol. 1984;74(1):26–33.
36. American College of Allergy, Asthma, & Immunology. Food allergy: a practice parameter. Ann Allergy Asthma Immunol. 2006;96(3 Suppl 2):S1–68.
37. Bernstein IL, Li JT, Bernstein DI, Hamilton R, Spector SL, Tan R, Sicherer S, Golden DB, Khan DA, Nicklas RA, Portnoy JM, Blessing-Moore J, Cox L, Lang DM, Oppenheimer J, Randolph CC, Schuller DE, Tilles SA, Wallace DV, Levetin E, Weber R, American Academy of Allergy, Asthma and Immunology, American College of Allergy, Asthma and Immunology. Allergy diagnostic testing: an updated practice parameter. Ann Allergy Asthma Immunol. 2008;100(3 Suppl 3):S1–148.
38. Kattan J, Sicherer S. Optimizing the diagnosis of food allergy. Immunol Allergy Clin N Am. 2015;35(1):61–76.
39. Čelakovská J, Krcmova I, Bukac J, Vaneckova J. Sensitivity and specificity of specific IgE, skin prick test and atopy patch test in examination of food allergy. Food Agric Immunol. 2016;28(2):238–47.
40. Ellis AK, Day JH. Incidence and characteristics of biphasic anaphylaxis: a prospective evaluation of 103 patients. Ann Allergy Asthma Immunol. 2007;98(1):64–9.
41. Sampson HA, Mendelson L, Rosen JP. Fatal and near-fatal anaphylactic reactions to food in children and adolescents. N Engl J Med. 1992;327(6):380–4.
42. Sheikh A, Ten Broek V, Brown SG, Simons FE. H1-antihistamines for the treatment of anaphylaxis: Cochrane systematic review. Allergy. 2007;62(8):830–7. Review.
43. Fedorowicz Z, van Zuuren EJ, Hu N. Histamine H2-receptor antagonists for urticaria. Cochrane Database Syst Rev. 2012;3:CD008596. https://doi.org/10.1002/14651858.CD008596.pub2. Review.
44. Choo KJ, Simons FE, Sheikh A. Glucocorticoids for the treatment of anaphylaxis. Evid Based Child Health. 2013;8(4):1276–94. https://doi.org/10.1002/ebch.1925. Review.
45. Douglas DM, Sukenick E, Andrade WP, Brown JS. Biphasic systemic anaphylaxis: an inpatient and outpatient study. J Allergy Clin Immunol. 1994;93(6):977–85.
46. Kemp SF. The post-anaphylaxis dilemma: how long is long enough to observe a patient after resolution of symptoms? Curr Allergy Asthma Rep. 2008;8(1):45–8. Review.
47. Cheng A. Emergency treatment of anaphylaxis in infants and children. Paediatr Child Health. 2011;16(1):35–40.
48. Mack DP. Biphasic anaphylaxis: a systematic review of the literature. Allergy Asthma Clin Immunol. 2014;10(Suppl 1):A5.
49. Clark S, Bock SA, Gaeta TJ, Brenner BE, Cydulka RK, Camargo CA, Multicenter Airway Research Collaboration-8 Investigators. Multicenter study of emergency department visits for food allergies. J Allergy Clin Immunol. 2004;113(2):347–52.
50. Arroabarren E, Lasa EM, Olaciregui I, Sarasqueta C, Muñoz JA, Pérez-Yarza EG. Improving anaphylaxis management in a pediatric emergency department. Pediatr Allergy Immunol. 2011;22(7):708–14. https://doi.org/10.1111/j.1399-3038.2011.01181.x. Epub 2011 Jun 15.
51. Campbell R, Li J, Nicklas R, Sadosty A. Emergency department diagnosis and treatment of anaphylaxis: a practice parameter. Ann Allergy Asthma Immunol. 2014;113(6):599–608.
52. Clark S, Long AA, Gaeta TJ, Camargo CA Jr. Multicenter study of emergency department visits for insect sting allergies. J Allergy Clin Immunol. 2005;116(3):643–9.

Early Recognition of Anaphylaxis in High Risk Settings

David R. Stukus

Fatal Anaphylaxis

In the United States, there are approximately 220 deaths from anaphylaxis each year, with a prevalence of 0.69 deaths per million persons [1]. Review of registry data offers an understanding of the common causes, which can help stratify risk. Unfortunately, registry records are often incomplete, with causes of anaphylaxis frequently not identified or listed. A large study published in 2014 identified 2458 deaths in the United States over an 11-year period and found that the majority of cases were caused by drugs, including radiocontrast media (59%), followed by venom (15%), and food allergies (7%) [1]. The ages of those affected varied significantly for each cause, with older adults much more likely to die from anaphylaxis overall, particularly due to medication and venom, compared with children and young adults. Interestingly, due to public interest and a robust engaging online food allergy community, anaphylaxis and rare reports of death from food allergies receive disproportionate attention in media reports and among patients and medical providers. By using data such as provided in this study, medical professionals can better educate patients and colleagues to understand that the majority of fatalities from anaphylaxis are actually caused by treatment interventions prescribed by healthcare professionals, such as medications and radiocontrast media. In addition to offering perspective and raising awareness, these discussions can redirect focus to the situations associated with highest risk.

While it is useful to understand that the general classification of "drugs" is the main cause for most fatal anaphylactic episodes, not all drugs are associated with the same high risk. Risk of severe reaction varies based upon frequency of use in the general population, method of administration, and structural properties of the drugs.

D. R. Stukus (✉)
Division of Allergy & Immunology, Nationwide Children's Hospital and The Ohio State College of Medicine, Columbus, OH, USA
e-mail: David.stukus@nationwidechildrens.org

© Springer Nature Switzerland AG 2020
A. K. Ellis (ed.), *Anaphylaxis*, https://doi.org/10.1007/978-3-030-43205-8_2

Antibiotics, muscle relaxants, chemotherapeutic agents, and radiocontrast media are the most common causes of fatal anaphylaxis [1, 2]. In addition, administration of a medication through the intravenous or intramuscular route is much more likely to cause anaphylaxis compared with oral or cutaneous exposure. Intravenous or muscular introduction can expose antigen to immunoglobulin E antibodies more rapidly and also activates other mediators involved in anaphylaxis such as the complement system, which can lead to a more rapid induction of a systemic allergic reaction.

Additional consideration should be given to symptoms that occur after administration of certain medications or transfusions which can mimic anaphylaxis and often involve the same mediators. Rapid administration of vancomycin can result in "red man syndrome" and associated flushing, itching, burning, and discomfort. Vancomycin is not a common allergen, but causes allergy types symptoms by direct mast cell and basophil stimulation. Unlike IgE-mediated drug allergy, patients who have experienced red man syndrome can receive vancomycin again by slowing the intravenous infusion rate and pretreatment with antihistamines. Another common cause of non-IgE-mediated symptoms that mimic anaphylaxis are radiocontrast media reagents. Many of these agents have a high osmolarity, which can cause direct mast cell and basophil degranulation through an osmolar effect achieved by rapid direct exposure through the venous circulation. Patients with a history of prior reactions to radiocontrast media can safely receive these agents again through well-established protocols that include use of low-osmolar agents and pretreatment with corticosteroids and antihistamines (Table 2.1) [3]. Opioids are a commonly used class of pain medications and have properties that can result in direct mast cell degranulation resulting in itching, urticaria, angioedema, and also anaphylaxis. True IgE-mediated allergic reactions to opioids are rare, and symptoms often improve by changing the dose, route of administration, or to a different class of analgesics.

While often reported and recorded on medical records as an "allergy," local anesthetics are very rare causes of IgE-mediated allergic reactions or anaphylaxis [4].

Table 2.1 Pretreatment regimens for patients with prior history of anaphylaxis to radiocontrast media

Nonurgent treatment	
Adult	Prednisone 50 mg at 13, 7, and 1 hour before procedure and diphenhydramine 50 mg 1 hour before procedure
Pediatric	Prednisone 0.5–0.7 mg/kg oral at 13, 7, and 1 hour before procedure and diphenhydramine 1.25 mg/kg 1 hour before the procedure
Emergency pretreatment	
Adult	Methylprednisolone 40 mg IV every 4 hours until procedure and diphenhydramine 50 mg IV 1 hour before contrast injection
Pediatric	Methylprednisolone 0.5 mg/kg IV every 4 hours until procedure and diphenhydramine 1.25 mg/kg 1 hour before contrast injection
	Lower/iso-osmolar radiocontrast media should be used in all cases when possible

The majority of reported systemic reactions from local anesthetics are non-allergic adverse effects caused by factors such as vagal activation, i.e., feeling lightheaded or experiencing syncope after receiving an injection prior to dental work or other medical procedures. As such, situations involving local anesthetics are associated with significantly less risk for anaphylaxis compared with other interventions such as intravenous administration of antibiotics.

Venom is the second most identified cause of fatal anaphylaxis [5]. Venom allergy will be covered in more detail elsewhere in this textbook, but basic concepts will be introduced at this time as they pertain to recognition of anaphylaxis in high-risk settings. Hymenoptera are the most likely causes of anaphylaxis from venom. These stinging insects include honey bees, yellow jackets, yellow hornets, white hornets, and wasps. Fire ants are another common cause of anaphylaxis from sting-ing insect but are isolated to certain geographic regions associated with year-round warmer climates. Risk for anaphylaxis from stinging insects varies based upon loca-tion, climate, and outdoor activities. Yellow jackets have been reported as the most likely cause of severe reactions and anaphylaxis, but any of these insects can cause a severe reaction.

While any food can potentially cause anaphylaxis, peanut and tree nuts are iden-tified as the cause of death for almost all severe reactions, particularly in teenagers and adults [6]. Milk, shellfish, and finned fish have also been reported to cause fatalities. While we want patients with other types of food allergy such as egg, wheat, or soy to follow successful avoidance strategies to prevent future reactions, it is important and helpful for people to understand that the risk for severe or life-threatening reactions from other foods differs from peanut and tree nuts. As dis-cussed further in this chapter, anxiety and poor quality of life from food allergies are an often-unrecognized consequence, which can dramatically impact a patient's life. As such, helping patients understand their risk in context of other food allergens can be a beneficial conversation.

Identifying Those at Risk

A clinical history of prior anaphylaxis and identification of IgE-mediated allergy toward the suspected cause is the best method to determine someone's future risk for anaphylaxis. Currently available skin prick and serum-specific IgE levels toward individual allergens cannot be used to indicate the severity of future reactions. Both skin prick and serum-specific IgE tests are useful in the evaluation of a patient who has a clinical history suggestive for IgE-mediated allergy [7]. However, both tests have high rates of false-positive results due to characteristics such as cross-reactivity with similar allergens, i.e., patients with birch tree pollen allergies may have an elevated peanut IgE test result even though they eat peanuts regularly without prob-lems. The low positive predictive value limits their ability to serve as screening tests, but both tests do offer high negative predictive value and can be useful in rul-ing out the presence of IgE-mediated allergy. IgE tests are too often reported or interpreted as "positive" or "negative" but this is a misinterpretation. The size of the

IgE test can only be used to determine the likelihood of IgE-mediated allergy being present, which must be interpreted in the context of the clinical history. Detectable IgE by skin prick or serum testing only indicates allergic sensitization and by itself is not diagnostic for allergy. A clinical history of rapid onset and/or recurrent symptoms consistent with an IgE-mediated allergy *and* detectable IgE through skin prick or serum testing is necessary to establish a diagnosis of allergy.

There are diagnostic tests in development that may better determine severity of future allergic reactions, but these are not currently validated or commercially available. One example is the basophil activation test, which is an in vitro test that measures markers of basophil activation after exposure to a patient's blood [8]. Larger responses to the assay are associated with more severe clinical symptoms. Another form of refined diagnostics includes component testing, which is becoming more widely available for food allergens, particularly peanut [9]. Individuals with peanut allergy can react to various specific antigens contained in peanut. Antigens are designated as Ara h 1, 2, 3, etc. Conventional skin prick or serum-specific IgE toward peanut can only detect the presence of IgE directed toward any one or combination of these specific antigens. However, component blood tests can evaluate each separate component of the peanut antigen profile and offer results to determine if a person has IgE directed toward antigens associated with clinical reactions, i.e., Ara h 1, 2, or 3, or toward antigens that cross-react with birch tree pollen and do not cause clinical symptoms with ingestion, i.e., Ara h 8. As with traditional IgE tests, component tests are often misinterpreted as indicating risk for anaphylaxis or severe reaction. However, component tests can only be utilized to indicate the likelihood of clinical reactivity compared with cross-reactivity in someone with allergic rhinitis caused by tree pollen. Thus, at this time, there are no diagnostic tests available to determine the severity of future allergic reactions.

As mentioned above, prior clinical history is the most reliable factor in determining future risk. Individuals with clear anaphylaxis from any exposure are at highest risk to develop anaphylaxis again with future exposure to that same, or similar, allergen. These patients warrant the most attention in regard to education surrounding future risk of anaphylaxis as well as management [10]. However, severe anaphylaxis can occur in patients who have had mild reactions previously or also as their initial presentation. Medication reactions may progress naturally over time, with changes in route of administration or in concordance with acute symptoms or inflammation from other causes that may be occurring at the time of administration. Venom reactions can progress naturally over time, become worse with multiple concurrent stings, or be more severe when other comorbid conditions are present, such as asthma or acute illness. Food allergy reactions can progress over time due to multiple factors, including type of food involved, quantity ingested, comorbid asthma (especially poorly controlled or symptomatic asthma), exercise, illness, stress, and stage of the menstrual cycle.

Individuals with a complex medical history and/or who have required frequent treatment with antibiotics or other medications are at elevated risk to experience adverse or allergic reactions with future exposure to medication (Table 2.2). Underlying atopy or prior history of medication allergies also increases risk for

Table 2.2 Factors that increase risk for severe or fatal anaphylaxis

Delayed administration of epinephrine
Age >65 years old
Underlying cardiovascular or pulmonary disease
Medication as the trigger
Use of β-blockers or ACE inhibitors
Uncontrolled asthma
Underlying mast cell disorder

anaphylaxis. Patients who are taking beta-blockers or angiotensin-converting enzyme inhibitors for the treatment of cardiovascular disease are at increased risk for severe anaphylaxis due to the inhibitory effect these medications have on the ability of epinephrine to act on beta-adrenergic receptors. Delayed administration of epinephrine is a common factor associated with cases of severe anaphylaxis and can be addressed through education, as discussed later in this chapter. Patients with underlying mast cell disorders such as systemic mastocytosis are at increased risk to have more severe symptoms during anaphylactic reactions [11]. Patients with selective IgA deficiency, defined as undetectable serum IgA levels (not simply lower than normal levels compared with laboratory reference ranges), have the potential to form anti-IgA IgE antibodies that can result in anaphylaxis from transfusions of various blood products, including whole blood and many IgG replacement products. Specific medication allergies are not inherited; thus, any parental self-report of reactions to specific medications has no impact on future generations and is not an indication to avoid that medication for the child or other family members.

Unfortunately, until a person is stung and experiences a systemic reaction, there is no current method to determine who may be at future risk from a severe allergic reaction from venom [5]. Venom allergy is not inherited; thus, any family members or parents who report their own history of severe allergy to stinging insects have no bearing on another individual. Prior history is the most important determining factor for who may be at risk for future anaphylaxis, and every patient who reports a suspected venom allergy or prior severe symptoms after a sting should have a detailed and thorough clinical history obtained. There are five types of symptoms that can occur after Hymenoptera stings and each determines future risk for anaphylaxis:

1. Local irritation, redness, itching, warmth, and swelling. This is a normal response to the toxins present in venom and does not increase risk for future reactions.
2. Diffuse cutaneous reactions in children <16 years of age. Generalized hives and itching without associated respiratory, gastrointestinal, or vascular symptoms after a sting in a child does not increase risk for anaphylaxis with future stings.
3. Diffuse cutaneous reactions in adults ≥16 years of age. Generalized hives and itching without associated respiratory, gastrointestinal, or vascular symptoms after a sting does, however, place adults at increased risk to experience anaphylaxis with future stings.
4. Large local reactions occur when a sting causes severe swelling, redness, and itching, confined to the same contiguous body part that was stung but without symptoms elsewhere. For example, a wasp sting on the wrist can cause severe

swelling of the hand or arm on the same side. These reactions also do not increase risk of anaphylaxis with future stings. There is a potential role for venom immunotherapy in patients who have frequent or severe discomfort from large local reactions, i.e., gardeners or landscapers.

5. Anaphylaxis. Prior history of rapidly progressive systemic reaction after a sting is the strongest risk factor for future anaphylaxis. Any patient who reports this type of reaction (careful review of medical records may be necessary to corroborate the history, particularly if symptoms occurred many years ago) warrants venom allergy testing and strong consideration for immunotherapy if elevated venom specific IgE is present. *These are the individuals that require the most education regarding their risk for anaphylaxis from future stings, including avoidance strategies and early recognition and treatment of anaphylaxis.*

Individuals with food allergies should be counseled about risk of reactions with future ingestion, but those with peanut, tree nut, seafood, and milk allergies (particularly toddlers and younger children) are at highest risk for future anaphylaxis. Those with underlying asthma should be counseled regarding the importance of adhering to a treatment plan in order to achieve good asthma control and prevent exacerbations. Anxiety is common among patients with food allergy and can become severe enough to decrease quality of life, interfere with social activities, and significantly impact the choices people make in regard to travel, dining out at restaurants, social gatherings, and participation in work/school activities. While all patients with food allergy should be counseled regarding the importance of avoiding accidental ingestion, including communication with all food handlers and reading labels on packaged products, and the importance of immediate access to their epinephrine autoinjector, not all patients have the same risk of anaphylaxis. Medical providers who diagnose or manage food allergies should routinely discuss quality of life, anxiety, and anticipatory guidance with every patient. For instance, it would be worthwhile to learn if a patient with egg allergy has not taken a vacation due to fear they will have inadvertent exposure to someone else's food containing egg as an ingredient while on a commercial airplane and then discuss the risks from these types of exposures and better address their anxiety. Likewise, it would be very worthwhile to learn of a patient with peanut allergy who never communicates with food handlers, does not routinely have access to their epinephrine autoinjector, and picks any nuts off their plate before eating, feeling that this is a "safe" practice. That patient may benefit from more education and understanding of their risky behavior.

Low Health Literacy

Health literacy is the degree to which individuals have the capacity to obtain, process, and understand basic health information needed to make appropriate health decisions. It is more than just reading ability. Unfortunately, only 12% of adults have proficient health literacy, which means almost 90% of adults lack skills needed to manage their health and prevent disease [12]. There are many factors that impact

Table 2.3 Factors the impact health literacy

Cultural background
Belief systems
Communication style
Complexity of information

Table 2.4 Steps to improve communication

Written information – use short words and sentences
Verbal communication – use simple, plain language and avoid jargon
Exhibit a general attitude of helpfulness
Review instructions and use the teach-back method
Speak slowly, pause, and allow time for and encourage questions
Utilize pictures, videos, and infographics to supplement written and verbal communication

an individual's level of health literacy and, in turn, how that impacts their personal care (Table 2.3). Patients with low health literacy are less likely to understand the signs and symptoms of anaphylaxis, know how and when to use epinephrine, and will be less equipped to avoid high-risk situations. Healthcare professionals must be aware of each individual patient's health literacy when discussing their care one-on-one in the healthcare setting, particularly when educating patients about anaphylaxis recognition and management.

There are readily available tools that medical professionals can utilize in the clinical setting to formally assess an individual's level of health literacy. However, these can be time-consuming and challenging to implement into routine practice. Fortunately, there are some basic techniques that providers can adopt to not only assess a patient's health literacy but also improve overall education and teaching practices (Table 2.4). An example of a simple method to improve communication is the teach-back method. When using the teach-back method, clinicians take the responsibility for adequate teaching and ask patients to repeat back or demonstrate what they were just taught. If patients are unable to adequately do so, the clinician takes the initiative to change their approach. This requires time and patience and is more successful if clinicians avoid any appearance of being rushed, annoyed, or bored. Most importantly, this forces clinicians to keep the information they provide simple, straightforward, and important.

Another example of a simple method to assess health literacy and improve communication are the Ask-Me-3 questions. The premise of Ask-Me-3 is to keep education simple and straightforward and also ensure that patients can answer three simple questions:

- What is my main problem?
- What do I need to do (about the problem)?
- Why is it important for me to do this?

If a patient can adequately answer these questions, they will have demonstrated knowledge pertaining to the most important aspects of their condition. For example, with anaphylaxis, a patient may reply "I could have a severe life-threatening reaction in the future. I need to avoid ____ and will do so by telling every waiter or waitress about my allergy and read all labels when I go shopping. I will make sure to always have my epinephrine in my bag/purse and with me at all times just in case I have any problems. This is important because if I can avoid ____ then I won't have any reactions and if I do have any problems, the earlier I use epinephrine, the better it works." Imagine if all of our patients could state that clearly at every visit.

Teenagers

If there is one age group or population that warrants the greatest attention in regard to anaphylaxis from food allergy, teenagers are by far at greatest risk [13]. While they are less likely to experience severe anaphylaxis or fatalities from drugs or venom, they are the age group to most likely experience fatalities from food allergy reactions. Central elements to the adolescent experience place them at greater risk for untoward outcomes, and it is important for medical providers to recognize and understand these factors and address them with their patients (and their parents).

Normal cognitive development during adolescence entails a transition from concrete thinking to more abstract thought processes and deeper appreciation for how our world operates and connects on various levels. The age at which this transition takes places varies considerably per individual, and some adults never fully achieve this transition or full cognitive development. Another key element of normal cognitive development for adolescents is an inability to understand and appreciate long-term consequences. They are simply incapable of anticipating how actions, or lack of action, in the present moment may lead to future consequences. In addition, risk taking is a normal part of adolescent growth and behavior. This is how adolescents learn to navigate the world and develop a sense of not only danger and boundaries but as much as possible at this stage consequences. When a lack of appreciation for long-term consequences is combined with a normal pattern of risk-taking behavior, we quickly understand why teenagers experiment with drugs, alcohol, and sexual activity. In regard to anaphylaxis, these are extremely important factors that parents and medical providers need to understand as it places teenagers at greater risk for severe outcomes.

There are a few scenarios that exemplify why teenagers are at highest risk for fatal food allergy reactions. They are less likely to have their epinephrine autoinjector available at all times and, even if available, are less likely to use it. Epinephrine is inconvenient to carry, to remember to take along when outside the home, and to use. Social encounters and peer support/pressure are generally the most important part of a teenager's life. Thus, anything that makes them stand out compared with their peers, seem different, or appear misunderstood can interfere with their self-management. Teens are more likely to eat a known food allergen when in a group setting even if they know it might make them sick and less likely to communicate with food handlers or notify their friends about their food allergy. When symptoms occur, they may not want to use their epinephrine as it may be embarrassing or necessitate the need to leave their social encounter to go to the hospital. Medical providers and parents can anticipate these common scenarios and discuss them with teenagers. In addition to describing why they are at increased risk for severe anaphylaxis, medical providers can offer practical tips to help them navigate these high-risk situations. By role-playing, practicing with training devices, and offering examples of effective communication skills, clinical encounters with teenagers can be useful learning experiences. But this cannot occur unless medical providers appreciate that teenagers at a high-risk cohort and actively address these issues during each encounter.

Early Recognition of Anaphylaxis

As discussed throughout this textbook, anaphylaxis is a rapidly progressive, systemic reaction that involves more than one organ system. Cutaneous symptoms such as urticaria, angioedema, and flushing occur in approximately 80% of cases of anaphylaxis [14]. However, absence of cutaneous symptoms does not exclude anaphylaxis and may portend a more severe reaction and lead to delayed administration of epinephrine. Gastrointestinal symptoms are more common among patients with known food allergies who experience anaphylaxis from accidental ingestion. Cardiovascular collapse and shock is a severe outcome and a contributing factor for fatal cases of medication and venom anaphylaxis in older adults. Clinical guidelines for the recognition of anaphylaxis designed for medical professionals list a provision for isolated hypotension as satisfying criteria for diagnosing anaphylaxis [14]. This will most likely present clinically in the specific scenario of an individual with known allergy who is knowingly exposed to their allergen. Practically, this will most commonly be encountered among patients with allergic rhinoconjunctivitis who are receiving subcutaneous immunotherapy injections in a physician's office. These patients can have more subtle signs of anaphylaxis, and given the recommended medical supervision for 30 minutes after each injection, subtle signs such as throat clearing, cough, nasal congestion, rhinorrhea, or lacrimation are more likely to be recognized early and prompt treatment.

For patients who have previously experienced anaphylaxis, it is important to review their prior reactions and help them understand what symptoms occurred so they can reference that experience in the future. While the same symptoms may not occur with future episodes, this is still a valuable learning exercise to help them pair their prior sensation with any future symptoms. It is also important to help patients understand the context in which anaphylaxis may occur. This is mostly based upon exposure to known allergens and will begin relatively soon afterward, often within minutes and rarely longer than 1–2 hours later. As discussed, patients with underlying allergic conditions are at risk to have anaphylaxis, but they will also have other allergy-related symptoms at other times. For example, it can be challenging for patients or parents of children at risk for anaphylaxis to distinguish urticaria during a viral infection from the initial manifestations of anaphylaxis. Other symptoms may mimic anaphylaxis as well (Table 2.5). Placing these symptoms in proper context of either the expected response from chronic allergic conditions, asthma, or chronic urticaria and common illnesses can help patients better understand when

Table 2.5 Situations that may mimic anaphylaxis

Cause	Symptoms
Asthma	Cough
	Wheeze
	Dyspnea
Vocal cord dysfunction	Acute onset stridor
	Dyspnea
Allergic rhinoconjunctivitis	Nasal congestion
	Sneezing
	Rhinorrhea
	Itching
Chronic urticaria	Exacerbation of underlying urticaria
Atopic dermatitis	Worsening rash after contact with irritant or allergen
Viral gastroenteritis	Acute onset emesis and/or diarrhea
Vasovagal syncope	Lightheadedness
	Syncope
	Feeling of impending doom
Contact urticaria/angioedema	Localized urticaria or angioedema

they should use epinephrine. Providing this anticipatory guidance can help patients better navigate future recognition and management of symptoms.

Location

Risk for anaphylaxis varies by location and according to trigger. Most cases of fatal anaphylaxis take place in the inpatient hospital setting or emergency department. This may be secondary to drugs being the main cause of fatal anaphylaxis, which are often administered intravenously in the hospital setting, which increases risk. It also may be related to patients admitted due to severe anaphylaxis and ultimately dying during that admission due to failure to improve with supportive care. Among those patients who suffer fatal reactions in the community setting before arrival to the hospital, this is most common in adults with venom-induced anaphylaxis and likely relates to stings occurring in locations a long distance from medical services, the rapid onset of symptoms associated with severe venom reactions, and delayed administration of epinephrine. Only 11% of fatalities from drugs, 13% from foods, and 18% from venom occurred outside the hospital setting in the large 2014 study of 2458 cases [1]. This information can be useful when educating medical providers who may be unaware of the much higher risk of severe anaphylaxis from medications in the hospital setting and also to help patients better understand and put their individual risk into proper context.

Hospital Setting

The perioperative setting is an area that warrants attention in regard to early recognition of anaphylaxis [3]. Antibiotics such as beta-lactams and neuromuscular blocking induction agents are some of the most common causes of medication-induced anaphylaxis and are also commonly used in the operating room. Symptoms from anaphylaxis can present at any time during an operation but often occur early and soon after intravenous administration of antibiotics or neuromuscular blocking agents, which are typically administered before the operation begins, although subsequent administration may occur throughout the case. Latex allergy has decreased markedly in recent years due to a major shift away from using latex gloves and products in most hospital settings. However, patients can still have latex allergy, particularly those with spina bifida or history of multiple operations or bladder catheterizations [15]. Frequent exposure of latex products to mucous membranes is a risk factor for developing latex allergy. As such, latex-induced anaphylaxis can occur in the peri-operative setting, and risk varies based upon patient background and type of instruments being used. Symptoms from latex-induced reactions may not occur until later in the course of the operation as exposure to vasculature or mucous membranes is the more typical inciting event for latex-induced anaphylaxis, as opposed to cutaneous exposure through skin or inhalation. Other rare considerations for causes of peri-operative anaphylaxis include induction agents such as propofol, sugammadex, or radiocontrast media.

Early recognition of anaphylaxis in the peri-operative setting can be challenging as patients are draped and their skin is obscured. As such, cutaneous symptoms, which are often the initial manifestation of anaphylaxis, are more likely to go unnoticed. More subtle signs such as acute difficulty with mechanical ventilation due to bronchoconstriction, tachycardia, and hypotension are more common initial signs in this setting. While all three of these signs can occur due to multiple events unrelated to anaphylaxis, any combination of these should raise immediate suspicion from the surgical team. Hypertension would be a rare sign of anaphylaxis as vasodilation is the expected vascular effect, leading to hypotension and tachycardia. Cases of suspected peri-operative anaphylaxis require careful scrutiny to determine if the timing of onset, type of exposure, and signs and symptoms are consistent with anaphylaxis and then to identify the potential cause. It can be useful to obtain a serum tryptase level when peri-operative anaphylaxis is suspected as acute elevation can support the clinical diagnosis and subsequent evaluation. Of note, the ideal time frame to draw a serum tryptase during suspected anaphylaxis from any cause is 1–4 hours after onset of initial symptoms. Outside of this time frame, including drawing a level too soon, can result in falsely negative results.

Routine childhood and adult vaccinations are typically administered in the medical setting. Anaphylaxis can occur and has been reported with most currently available vaccines, but it is important for both medical providers and patients to understand that this is an extremely rare occurrence. A 2016 study identified a rate of anaphylaxis from vaccine administration at 1.31 cases per million doses administered [16]. IgE-mediated reactions to vaccines can be caused by various vaccine components, which vary by individual vaccine and can include the antigen, food components such as gelatin, antibiotics, and other preservatives. Egg allergy is often misconstrued as a contraindication to administration of the measles-mumps-rubella (MMR) vaccine or seasonal influenza vaccine as these are cultured in hen's embryos, which theoretically could introduce minute amounts of egg protein into the vaccine. However, multiple studies and clinical guidelines stipulate that there is no increased risk for IgE-mediated reaction to either the MMR or influenza vaccine in patients who have a history of egg allergy, including anaphylaxis to egg [16]. There is no indication to perform any testing prior to administration or take any special precautions as these vaccines do not contain enough egg to provoke a reaction or it is not present in a form that can readily bind to IgE. While medical providers should be aware that allergic reactions can occur very rarely after vaccine administration, they can be reassured regarding the overall safety of vaccines in this regard.

Home

While <10% of deaths from anaphylaxis occur inside the home, anaphylactic reactions occur much more frequently and warrant attention in this setting. Food allergens are the most likely cause of anaphylaxis at home, and patients should be counseled regarding best practices to help reduce accidental ingestion. The main challenge occurs when one member of a household is allergic to a specific food, or foods, which other members of the house continue to consume that food(s) inside the home. Casual exposure to dust from food allergens, airborne particles, or proximity during cooking is very unlikely to cause anaphylaxis. The one exception is stove top heating or steaming of a few specific allergens such as shellfish, finned fish, or milk, which can aerosolize food proteins and cause asthma or respiratory symptoms in allergic individuals; however, this is a rare occurrence. Families should be counseled that they can safely have food allergens present inside the home and prevent food allergy reactions from occurring in affected individuals, which is particularly important for ubiquitous allergens such as milk, egg, wheat, and soy. As such, the focus for patients or parents of food-allergic children should center on preventing accidental ingestion.

Accidental ingestion of known food allergens inside the home can occur in various scenarios:

- Not reading labels on packaged products that contain allergen. Labels and ingredients can change without any notification from the manufacturer; thus, labels should be read carefully before every purchase and consumption.
- Cross contact of allergen can occur through shared utensils. Separate utensils are ideal when preparing a meal or snack for a food-allergic individual, but their meals can also be prepared first, then placed in a separate location. Soap and water, or washing through a dishwasher, can effectively remove food allergens from surfaces, utensils, and cooking equipment. In addition, commercial detergent wipes can also remove proteins from surfaces and tabletops but hand sanitizers, anti-bacterial gels, and water alone are not effective in this regard.
- Misidentification of safe foods. Families who have to avoid multiple food allergens or households with multiple affected individuals may be challenged in finding safe storage locations and keeping items separate. Creating a labeling system with clear demarcation and bright colors can prevent misidentification.
- Multiple caregivers, babysitters, and social gatherings also create challenges. Preparation and availability of safe food alternatives can help prevent exclusion

and confusion from those who are not versed on the necessity of food allergen avoidance. Parents of food-allergic children are often responsible for educating others regarding their child's food allergy, and medical providers can assist them with talking points and important areas to discuss. A general approach could include an example such as:

My child is allergic to ___ food(s). If they accidentally eat even small amounts of their allergen, it could make them very sick. We can avoid accidents by reading all labels very carefully and making sure that their meals or snacks do not touch their allergen at any time, including through shared utensils or cooking equipment. There are many safe foods they can eat, which we have prepared and labeled clearly. Symptoms of an allergic reaction usually start very soon after ingestion and can include itching, hives, skin rash, swelling, vomiting, or difficulty breathing. Here is their food allergy treatment plan, which outlines exactly what to do in case symptoms occur. This is their epinephrine autoinjector, which should be used as soon as possible if they are having anaphylaxis – it will not hurt them if used by mistake or if you are not sure, but not using it could cause their reaction to become very severe. Here's a training device that you can practice with to get used to how it works. If epinephrine is given, then you should call 911 as they will need to be monitored in case symptoms return or do not improve. I realize this may seem like a lot to take in, but once you get used to double-checking all food choices and focusing on preventing accidental ingestion, anyone can successfully follow food allergen avoidance. What questions do you have?

While medication-induced anaphylaxis can also occur at home, this is much less frequent than in the hospital setting. However, patients with prior anaphylaxis to medications should be counseled regarding how many pills look alike and have similar names. Any concern for cross-reactivity should be discussed as well, i.e., patients with allergy to non-steroidal anti-inflammatory medications must understand the similarities between ibuprofen and Naprosyn but safety with acetaminophen.

Severe reactions from venom often occur near the home, and avoidance measures are paramount for anyone with a prior history of anaphylaxis. Patients should be counseled to never walk outdoors in bare feet to avoid accidentally stepping on a honey bee, hornet, wasp, or yellow jacket. Beverages should never be consumed from cans or any container that occludes visibility to prevent accidentally swallowing a stinging insect. Many hymenoptera are drawn to perfumes, colognes, and bright colors, and these should be avoided when outdoors. Wasps, yellow jackets, and hornets are foragers, attracted to garbage collection areas, picnics, and any open food sources. They can become particularly aggressive in the late summer and autumn. Lastly, patients should be advised to actively avoid any known hives or nests and to use professional extermination services for removal.

Restaurants

Food allergies are the main concern for patients at risk for anaphylaxis dining at restaurants. Patients with food allergies can safely dine at restaurants but must learn and employ new communication skills. Calling ahead to discuss allergen avoidance practices can be helpful in making safe choices regarding destination. Upon arrival to a restaurant, the need to avoid specific allergens should be actively discussed with the waiter or waitress, who should then discuss with the chef. Many restaurants are becoming more educated and accommodating for customers with food allergies, and chefs will often come to the table to discuss safe preparation and optimal food choices given their knowledge of the menu and cooking practices. There are examples of food allergen identification and communication cards that can be handed out to restaurant personnel and outline the need to avoid specific allergens and risks of ingestion. This approach can be particularly useful when traveling abroad as they can be translated into different languages and help reduce risk for miscommunication.

Risk for accidental ingestion of a food allergen at a restaurant varies by allergen and type of food offerings. Asian restaurants present higher risk for peanut and tree nut exposure given their wide use of these ingredients in their menu items. Buffet lines can be risky due to cross contact from shared utensils and misidentification of food items. Bakeries that use peanuts, tree nuts, or other allergens may introduce exposure through cross contact by using the same baking sheet, food preparation area, or utensils. Ice cream parlors also have higher risk due to multiple flavors, wide-ranging ingredients, and shared use of scoopers that are often "cleaned" by dipping in water without soap. A common misconception relates to the safety of peanut oil for peanut-allergic individuals. Most restaurants use commercial grade peanut oil, which is highly refined and does not contain peanut protein, making it safe for ingestion. However, cold pressed and unrefined peanut oil (which is generally much more expensive and less utilized in restaurants) can contain peanut protein and provoke a reaction with ingestion. By focusing on specific scenarios such as these, patients can be counseled specifically regarding their personal allergens and high-risk situations when dining away from home. Lastly, patients should be reminded to always have their epinephrine autoinjectors with them at all times when dining out in case of accidental ingestion.

Schools

Food allergies are the main consideration for risk for anaphylaxis in the school setting, although children or school personnel with history of venom anaphylaxis must exercise caution when outdoors or near landscaping. Food allergy management in the school is complicated by the large number of students, challenges that prevent direct supervision at all times, consumption of food and snacks in the classroom and lunchroom, education level and comfort of teachers and school personnel, and various ages of students. Toddlers in the preschool setting require more direct supervision and consideration for a more careful environmental assessment given the normal developmental use of their mouths and hands when exploring their environment. Teenagers in high school are at risk for intentional ingestion and lack of preparedness, as discussed previously in this chapter.

Ideally, every child with a food allergy should have their personal epinephrine autoinjector available at school and an updated food allergy treatment plan filled out by their physician and shared with the school every year. There are excellent resources that discuss safe approaches to caring for all students with food allergy and are available to be shared with schools, including the free Voluntary

Guidelines for Management of Food Allergies in Schools and Early Care and Education Programs that was published by the Centers for Disease Control and Prevention in 2013 [17]. A recent phenomenon occurring in schools involves the adoption of nut-free policies. These are nebulous declarations designed to address concerns from parents of nut-allergic children and protect them from accidental ingestion and environmental exposure. There are both pros and cons to this approach that each school should consider prior to enacting such policies. There is no evidence that demonstrates any benefit from such bans, and interestingly, there is evidence from a study looking at over 1000 Massachusetts schools that epinephrine usage for the treatment of anaphylaxis was higher in schools which proclaimed themselves to be "nut-free" [18]. The number of school buildings, size of each building, physical layout, availability of adult supervision, presence or absence of a full-time school nurse, policies surrounding food-free class-rooms, age of students, and other factors should all be considered under reasons to think about implementing a nut-free policy. Downsides and unintentional con-sequences must also be considered in any thoughtful discussion surrounding nut-free polices, which includes the inability for any school to enforce a nut-free policy to any great extent as this would require daily inspection and reading labels of all food brought into the school by every child and school personnel. In addition, nut-free polices do not protect children with other common food aller-gies such as milk, egg, wheat, or seafood and may alienate those children and parents. Lastly, parents and school personnel may lessen their attention to chil-dren with peanut and tree nut allergies when nut-free policies are in place due to a false sense of security. This may lead to less availability of epinephrine or delayed recognition of symptoms.

Educating Those at Risk

Several important points of emphasis were discussed earlier in this chapter regard-ing how to best educate patients and medical professionals surrounding anaphy-laxis, early recognition of symptoms, and high-risk situations. Patients at risk for future anaphylaxis should all be educated regarding what allergens they need to avoid, the signs and symptoms of anaphylaxis, and indications for using epineph-rine. In addition, proper technique for epinephrine autoinjectors should be reviewed and practiced at every clinical encounter, ideally with the aid of a needleless training device. Hands-on training allows patients to practice each step and for constructive criticism to occur. At the time of this publication, three different epinephrine auto-injectors were commercially available in the United States, and each required differ-ent technique for proper administration. As such, individual devices should be reviewed and practiced, depending upon which type is prescribed (which may vary based upon patient preference, availability, and insurance coverage).

This chapter also reviewed other factors that warrant individual attention and discussion regarding increased risk for more severe anaphylaxis. Patients with underlying asthma, with medication and venom allergies, with advanced age, and who are taking beta-blockers or ACE inhibitors should have special attention regarding these risk factors and discussion of how best to mitigate risk for each circumstance. However, there is one risk factor associated with almost all cases of fatal anaphylaxis in the community setting which is fortunately amenable to education and preparation: delayed administration of epinephrine.

There are many reasons why epinephrine is routinely not administered for the treatment of anaphylaxis, including many misconceptions surrounding its use [19]. Although epinephrine is well established as the only effective first-line treatment for anaphylaxis, it is underutilized by patients, emergency responders, and even emergency room physicians. This extremely important discussion point should be emphasized with all patients and medical providers who care for patients with anaphylaxis. Table 2.6 summarizes key discussion points that relate

Table 2.6 Contributing factors to delayed administration of epinephrine for the treatment of anaphylaxis

Contributing factor	Discussion point
Patient-related factors	
High cost of epinephrine	Prescribe alternate device
	Ensure patients are aware of options
	Online coupons, patient assistance programs
Lack of availability once prescribed	Discuss importance of immediate access to devices in all situations
	Role-play; discuss specific methods to improve carriage rates
Lack of use even when available	Discuss safety, efficacy, and importance of using early
	Give clear indications for use
	Review benefit of using even if not necessary is greater than risk of not using when anaphylaxis occurs
Incorrect technique	Review with training device at each clinical encounter
	Anticipate common errors to discuss: not removing cap, holding wrong end, not injecting into thigh, not holding for pre-specified time
Physician-related factors	
Missed diagnosis	Education regarding proper interpretation of IgE tests and clinical history
Lack of epinephrine prescriptions	Ensure prescriptions for all patients deemed at risk for anaphylaxis
Lack of specialist referral	Allergists should be consulted (when available and feasible) for patients at high risk for anaphylaxis to assist in diagnosis and management
General misconceptions	
Epinephrine is dangerous	When administered in dosages found in autoinjectors and through proper intramuscular injection, cardiac complications are very rare
	Intravenous administration or through boluses are the situations associated with risk for cardiac complications
	Lacerations are infrequent adverse effects but can be prevented through proper technique
Emergency room evaluation is necessary due to danger of epinephrine	Epinephrine is safe in doses provided in autoinjectors and transport to nearest emergency room is for evaluation in case epinephrine wears off or symptoms return
	Patients may be reluctant to use epinephrine as they do not want to interrupt their current engagement to go to the emergency room; these patients may benefit from a plan that allows for close monitoring after epinephrine is used and transport only if symptoms do not improve

to delayed administration of epinephrine. Medical professionals can use these as talking points to educate patients and review at each visit. Each topic may not apply to all individuals but collectively represent some of the most common areas of misunderstanding.

Conclusion

Early recognition and treatment of anaphylaxis is important to optimize patient outcomes. Through use of registry data surrounding fatalities from anaphylaxis and understanding risk factors involved with the most severe cases, medical professionals can identify and help educate patients at high risk for severe anaphylaxis. The inpatient setting warrants the greatest attention due to potential for severe anaphylaxis from medications and radiocontrast media. Proper diagnosis of patients with medication, venom, and food allergies and education regarding avoidance are the first steps involved at protecting patients at highest risk for severe anaphylaxis. Anticipatory guidance, role-playing, practicing with epinephrine autoinjector training devices, and discussion of common misconceptions and scenarios surrounding delayed administration of epinephrine are all important areas of discussion to focus on during clinical encounters.

References

1. Jerschow E, Lin RY, Scaperotti MM, McGinn AP. Fatal anaphylaxis in the United States, 1999-2010: temporal patterns and demographic associations. J Allergy Clin Immunol. 2014;134:1318–28.
2. Turner PJ, Jerschow E, Umasunthar T, Lin R, Campbell DE, Boyle RJ. Fatal anaphylaxis: mortality rate and risk factors. J Allergy Clin Immunol Pract. 2017;5:1169–78.
3. Blatman KS, Hepner DL. Current knowledge and management of hypersensitivity to perioperative drugs and radiocontrast media. J Allergy Clin Immunol Pract. 2017;5:587–92.
4. Boren E, Teuber SS, Naguwa SM, Gershwin ME. A critical review of local anesthetic sensitivity. Clin Rev Allergy Immunol. 2007;32(1):119–28.
5. Golden DBK, Demain J, Freeman T, Graft D, Tankersley M, Tracy J, et al. Stinging insect hypersensitivity: a practice parameter update 2016. Ann Allergy Asthma Immunol. 2017;118:28–54.
6. Bock SA, Munoz-Furlong A, Sampson HA. Further fatalities caused by anaphylactic reactions to food, 2001–2006. J Allergy Clin Immunol. 2007;119(4):1016–8.
7. Sampson HA, Aceves S, Bock SA, James J, Jones S, Lang D, et al. Food allergy: a practice parameter update-2014. J Allergy Clin Immunol. 2014;134(5):1016–25.
8. Santos AF, Shreffler WG. Road map for the clinical application of the basophil activation test in food allergy. Clin Exp Allergy. 2017;47(9):1115–24.
9. Klemans RJ, van Os-Mendendorp H, Blankestijn M, Bruijnzeel-Koomen CA, Knol EF, Knulst AC. Diagnostic accuracy of specific IgE to components in diagnosing peanut allergy: a systematic review. Clin Exp Allergy. 2015;45(4):720–30.
10. Golden DBK. Anaphylaxis: recognizing risk and targeting treatment. J Allergy Clin Immunol Pract. 2017;5(5):1224–6.
11. Gülen T, Ljung C, Nilsson G, Akin C. Risk factor analysis of anaphylactic reactions in patients with systemic mastocytosis. J Allergy Clin Immunol Pract. 2017;5:1248–55.
12. Rudd RE. Health literacy: insights and issues. Stud Health Technol Inform. 2017;240:60–78.

13. Stukus DR, Nassef M, Rubin M. Leaving home: helping teens with allergic conditions become independent. Ann Allergy Asthma Immunol. 2016;116(5):388–91.
14. Sampson HA, Munoz-Furlong A, Campbell RL, Adkinson NF, Bock SA, Branum A, et al. Second symposium on the definition and management of anaphylaxis: summary report—Second National Institute of Allergy and Infectious Disease/Food Allergy and Anaphylaxis Network symposium. J Allergy Clin Immunol. 2006;117:391–7.
15. Kelly KJ, Sussman G. Latex allergy: where are we now and how did we get there? J Allergy Clin Immunol Pract. 2017;5:1212–6.
16. Greenhawt M, Turner PJ, Kelso JM. Administration of influenza vaccines to egg allergic recipients: a practice parameter update 2017. Ann Allergy Asthma Immunol. 2018;120(1):49–52.
17. Centers for Disease Control and Prevention. Voluntary guidelines for managing food allergies in schools and early care and education programs. Washington, D.C.: US Department of Health and Human Services; 2013. Available at: www.cdc.gov/HealthyYouth/foodallergies/pdf/13_243135_A_Food_Allergy_Web_508.pdf. Last accessed on 17 Jan 2019.
18. Bartnikas LM, Huffaker MF, Sheehan WJ, Kanchongkittiphon W, Petty CR, Leibowitz R, et al. Impact of school peanut-free policies on epinephrine administration. J Allergy Clin Immunol. 2017;140:465–73.
19. Prince BT, Mikhail I, Stukus DR. Underuse of epinephrine for the treatment of anaphylaxis: missed opportunities. J Asthma Allergy. 2018;11:143–51.

Management of Anaphylaxis Refractory to Standard First Line Therapy

3

Catherine Hammond and Jay Lieberman

The term anaphylaxis (Greek for "opposite protection") was first coined by Charles Richet and Paul Portier in 1901 as a result of their work attempting to immunize dogs to sea anemone toxin. Rather than immunizing the dogs, they caused a hypersensitivity reaction upon re-exposure to the toxin and thus coined the term to suggest they provided the opposite of prophylaxis, or anaphylaxis. In the over 100 years following this initial description, our knowledge of the causes and pathophysiology of anaphylaxis has expanded greatly. However, despite over a century of research into the phenomenon, there is still controversy surrounding the precise definition of the term, leading to inconsistent diagnosis and treatment [1]. In fact, most organizations around the world still have their own definition of anaphylaxis, none of which use the exact same terminology [2–4]. In response to the lack of uniformity in definition, the National Institute of Allergy and Infectious Disease (NIAID) and the Food Allergy and Anaphylaxis Network (FAAN) convened a panel of experts to establish clinically relevant criteria to aid in the management of anaphylaxis [5]. The results of this discussion provided clinical criteria for when anaphylaxis is likely, namely, when one of the following occurs: (1) acute onset of an illness with generalized skin or mucosal involvement with flushing, hives, or pruritus; (2) acute cutaneous, cardiorespiratory, or gastrointestinal symptoms after exposure to a likely allergen; and (3) acute reduction of blood pressure after exposure to a known allergen. The point of these criteria was not to provide a definition of anaphylaxis, but rather to provide clinicians scenarios for which administration of epinephrine is appropriate. This is paramount, as no matter the definition used, epinephrine is the agreed-upon first-line treatment for anaphylaxis. In most scenarios, epinephrine and supportive measures will allow for resolution of symptoms. However, there are clearly cases in which the reaction is refractory to epinephrine.

C. Hammond · J. Lieberman (✉)
Department of Pediatrics, Allergy/Immunology, University of Tennessee Health Science Center, Memphis, TN, USA
e-mail: chammo17@uthsc.edu; jlieber1@uthsc.edu

© Springer Nature Switzerland AG 2020
A. K. Ellis (ed.), *Anaphylaxis*, https://doi.org/10.1007/978-3-030-43205-8_3

The purpose of this chapter is to review current literature and assemble information on the epidemiology, risk factors, prevention, and treatment of refractory anaphylaxis as well as discuss potential areas for future research.

Definition and Epidemiology

Given the variability and lack of unified definition of anaphylaxis, it is easy to understand that there is no single accepted definition of refractory anaphylaxis. One review of case reports chose to define refractory anaphylaxis as anaphylaxis (meeting NIAID/FAAN criteria) "unresponsive to the treatment with at least two doses of a minimum 300 micrograms adrenaline" (with unresponsiveness being defined as "a lack of expected normalization of clinical symptoms") [6]. Alternatively, when referring to perioperative anaphylaxis, one proposed definition is persistent severe shock after 10 minutes of adequate resuscitation [7].

Prevalence of anaphylaxis has been difficult to ascertain and has been estimated to be somewhere between 0.3% and 5.1% depending on the geographic location, definition used, age, and setting (emergency department, hospitalization, etc.) sampled and appears to be increasing in most series, with a concomitant increase in fatal anaphylactic reactions [8, 9]. In addition, there is evidence to suggest that the condition is underdiagnosed [10]. Unfortunately, there is no series that has attempted to define the frequency of refractory anaphylaxis among patients with anaphylaxis. There are reports to at least suggest that the majority of the cases of refractory anaphylaxis is associated with intraoperative anaphylaxis, suggesting this may be a risk factor for refractory anaphylaxis [6]. However, this may simply be due to the fact that during intraoperative anaphylaxis, the patients are already under medical care when the reactions occurs and thus receive early treatment and are able to be classified as "refractory" when the treatment fails, whereas patients who have severe reactions "in the field" that would be classified as refractory end up not getting therapy early or at all and thus end up being classified as fatal or near-fatal reactions, rather than refractory.

Risk Factors

There are several published case series of severe, near-fatal, and fatal anaphylaxis. While these have not specifically examined "refractory" anaphylaxis, the severity of these cases suggest that they would likely be patients refractory to treatment in many cases, and thus examining these case series can help shed light on risk factors for refractory anaphylaxis [11–16]. In fact, in many of these cases, epinephrine was administered, but did not resolve the symptoms. One must understand however that the risk factors are likely to be dependent on the trigger (food, venom, medication, etc.) and age of the cohort studied. For example, in examining all patients presenting to an emergency department with anaphylaxis, Motosue et al. showed that risks for severe anaphylaxis (defined admission to hospital or intensive care unit, requiring endotracheal intubation, or meeting criteria for a near-fatal reaction) included age of 65 or older, anaphylaxis triggered by medication, and underlying cardiac or lung disease [11]. However, when examining only select triggers of anaphylaxis, the risk factors may change. For fatal anaphylaxis caused by drugs (which is most commonly due to beta-lactam antibiotics, general anesthetic agents, or radiocontrast media), older age and underlying cardiovascular disease continue to show associations with severe anaphylaxis. For anaphylaxis due to foods only however, delayed epinephrine administration, age in the second or third decade of life, concomitant asthma, and nut allergy (peanuts and tree nuts) have all been associated with fatal reactions in various case series [13, 14, 16]. In contrast, in a large series of pediatric anaphylaxis cases in Europe, when teasing out triggers for severe and fatal reactions, the triggers were no different than the spectrum of foods that triggered all cases of anaphylaxis [17]. Thus, defining risk factors for severe or refractory anaphylaxis is difficult and must be discussed in the context of trigger and possibly age.

In general, delayed administration of epinephrine has been linked to refractoriness to treatment and to mortality [18–20]. This once again likely relates to the fact that severe and fatal anaphylaxis episodes may possibly be reclassified as "refractory" if treated early with epinephrine, as these episodes would likely require more intense treatment.

When specifically examining cases of refractory anaphylaxis, risk factors tend to be similar to the abovementioned associations; however, because many of these cases are medically monitored, risk factors can be viewed with slightly greater granularity. For example, a recent review article of 151 cases of refractory anaphylaxis identified several patient-dependent and iatrogenic factors that may contribute to refractory anaphylaxis. Patient-dependent factors included impaired right ventricular function, coronary artery disease, older age, and bronchial hyperresponsiveness, while iatrogenic factors included failure to cease allergen exposure, late epinephrine injection, insufficient volume resuscitation, and concomitant beta-blocker use [6].

This same review found that the vast majority (73.8%) of cases occurred perioperatively [6]. Specifically, those patients concomitantly undergoing treatment with protamine-containing insulins had a significantly higher (up to 40–50 times greater) risk of perioperative refractory anaphylaxis [21]. While an interesting observation, this patient population already represents a unique subset of anaphylaxis cases given the difficulty of diagnosing anaphylaxis perioperatively (due to patient inability to communicate subjective symptoms and surgical drapes hiding cutaneous symptoms) as well as mechanism of exposure (typically intravenous) [22].

Future studies further investigating the risk factors for refractory anaphylaxis would be useful both to identify patients at risk prior to their potential exposures and to treat patients with risk factors who experience anaphylaxis more aggressively earlier.

Prevention

Prevention of refractory anaphylaxis follows the same tenets of prevention of anaphylaxis in general. First and foremost is identifying patients at risk for anaphylaxis. Current guidelines are in place to aid in the diagnosis and prevention of anaphylaxis.

Understanding factors associated with refractory anaphylaxis as mentioned above though can help to identify patients who are more at risk for severe reactions and thus patients who need closer attention. For patients with food allergy, for example, special attention should be paid to optimizing asthma management and educating adolescents on risk-taking behaviors.

There is no pharmacologic management currently available to use as prophylaxis to prevent anaphylaxis or to make reactions less severe. Interestingly though, there are case reports of omalizumab showing its success in anaphylaxis prophylaxis in certain populations, including idiopathic anaphylaxis and mastocytosis/mast cell activation syndrome [23]. There are case reports showing success of omalizumab in preventing episodes of anaphylaxis in patients (both pediatric and adult) with idiopathic anaphylaxis [24–27]. In addition, there have also been reports of omalizumab preventing anaphylaxis in pediatric [28, 29] and adult patients [30–33] with systemic mastocytosis or mast cell activation syndrome. Though these are case reports rather than large formal trials, it does suggest that omalizumab may be useful in the prevention of anaphylaxis and could perhaps be useful in patients with a history of refractory anaphylaxis as well.

Treatment

Traditional Considerations for First-Line Agents

Most important in the treatment of any case of anaphylaxis is early administration of epinephrine. Although never formally studied in a randomized controlled trial (for obvious ethical and logistical reasons), there is enough evidence that expert guidelines all agree that it is the most important first-line life-saving treatment [1–5]. Other medications often given early in anaphylaxis include corticosteroids and antihistamines. No randomized controlled trials on the effectiveness of corticosteroids in anaphylaxis have been conducted, but two recent large scale reviews failed to show strong support for their routine use [34, 35]. In addition, corticosteroids do not seem to be helpful in the prevention of biphasic anaphylaxis [36]. Similarly, there are no randomized controlled trials on effectiveness of antihistamines for the treatment of anaphylaxis. Nevertheless, these classes of medications are still often used for initial treatment of anaphylaxis, and in some emergency departments, they are used more often than epinephrine for anaphylaxis [17, 37–39]. Based on the recommendations of the most recent practice parameter, these medications can be considered for optional adjunctive therapy but are not indicated as initial treatment [3]. It would be reasonable, then, to also consider their use in cases of refractory anaphylaxis as well, though never to delay administration of epinephrine.

Traditional Considerations for Second-Line Agents

When anaphylaxis is refractory to epinephrine, additional measures should be taken in hopes to prevent cardiovascular shock and/or respiratory arrest. These actions are likely to be done simultaneously and should be considered in any case of anaphylaxis; however, in cases refractory to epinephrine, there is little to no reason for these not to be attempted.

Perhaps the easiest measure to be done is placing the patient in a supine position (or on the left side in the case of pregnant patients). Past recommendations have supported placing the legs above the head or in Trendelenburg position; however, the most recent American guidelines discuss that this is controversial given limited evidence to support its use and some possible unintended consequences [3, 40]. If possible, oxygen should be administered. While there are no studies designed to specifically examine oxygen and goal saturations, it is reasonable to titrate the oxygen for saturations of 94–96% by oximetry. Also, if available, intravenous access should be obtained and volume replacement administered if indicated [41].

Additional pharmacologic measures to consider in the treatment of refractory anaphylaxis at this stage include second-line agents (if not given already) such as β2-agonists, H1 and H2 antihistamines, and corticosteroids. Antihistamines and corticosteroids (as mentioned above) are not likely to affect outcomes in anaphylaxis; however, there is little downside to administering these medications as further interventions are being undertaken in refractory cases. Example doses for these are given in Table 3.1 (these doses are mainly anecdotal and drawn for their use in other conditions, as no dose ranging studies have been carried out in anaphylaxis). Inhaled β2-agonists arguably have a more important role in refractory anaphylaxis than antihistamines and corticosteroids. As discussed above, asthma is a risk factor for severe reactions, especially for food-induced reactions. Thus, based on this and the quick onset of action for β2-agonists, it is reasonable to administer β2-agonists while other steps are being taken to stabilize and treat refractory cases. In fact, in early case series of food-induced fatal anaphylaxis reactions, investigators felt that asthma and bronchoconstriction led to respiratory failure and death and suggested that administration of β2-agonists in these cases may be as important as administration of epinephrine [42, 43].

Finally, additional doses of IM epinephrine should be given in cases of refractory anaphylaxis as the patient is being stabilized. Interestingly, whether given by auto-injector or utilizing doses drawn up by medical professionals, epinephrine is often given in error (e.g., incorrect location, incorrect dose, or incorrect route), and thus one should always ensure that the appropriate dose of epinephrine was administered in the appropriate location [44–46]. If appropriate dose and administration has been ensured and the patient still shows a lack of response, one should consider repeating appropriate dose. One study of pharmacokinetics of the available 0.3 mg epinephrine autoinjections (EpiPen and Auvi-Q) found that both products reach maximum plasma concentration most often within 3–9 minutes; however, a small percentage of patients took much longer, up to 1 hour, to achieve maximum plasma concentration. Half-life was also similar between the two products and ranged from 60 to 90 minutes among participants [47]. Based on these data, it would be reasonable to

Table 3.1 Second-line agents for anaphylaxis

Second-line agents for anaphylaxis treatment	Refractory anaphylaxis review article suggested dose [1]	Anaphylaxis practice parameter suggested dose [2]	Comments
Oxygen	Initiate early, titrate according to clinical response and device used	6–10 L/min, up to 100%	Titrate to oxygen saturations 94–96%
Fluid replacement	Adult: 1–2 L normal saline IV rapidly; *or* Ringer's lactate 5–10 mL/ kg in the first 5 minutes Pediatric: 20 mL/kg Ringer's lactate in the first hour	Adult: 1–2 L normal saline IV rapidly Pediatric: up to 30 mL/kg IV normal saline in the first hour	Monitor for signs of volume overload
β2-Agonists	Albuterol via nebulization with oxygen (no dosages specified)	Adult: 2.5–5 mg/3 mL of saline nebulized albuterol Pediatric: 2.5 mg/3 mL saline of nebulized albuterol	
Antihistamines H1 blockers	Adult: IV diphenhydramine 25–50 mg over 10 minutes Pediatric: IV diphenhydramine 1 mg/kg (up to 50 mg) over 10 minutes	Adult: IV diphenhydramine 25–50 mg over 10–15 minutes Pediatric: IV diphenhydramine 1 mg/kg (up to 50 mg) over 10–15 minutes	Should not be used as substitute for epinephrine
H2 blockers	Adult: IV ranitidine 50 mg over 10 minutes Pediatric: IV ranitidine 12.5–50 mg over 10 minutes	Adult: 1 mg/kg IV ranitidine via slow infusion Pediatric: 12.5–50 mg IV ranitidine via slow infusion	
Corticosteroids	IV methylprednisolone 1–2 mg/kg/day; OR PO prednisone 0.5 mg/kg/day	1–2 mg/kg per dose up to 125 mg methylprednisolone or an equivalent formulation	Should not be used as substitute for epinephrine
Glucagon	Initial dose of 1–5 mg slow IV and then 5–15 μg/ min infusion	Adult: 1–5 mg IV over 5 minutes and then 5–15 μg/min infusion Pediatric: 20–30 mg/kg IV (maximum 1 mg) IV over 5 minutes and then 5–15 μg/min infusion	Can cause emesis, considered airway protection (especially in obtunded patient)
Positioning	Not mentioned	Supine position	Pregnant patient in left lateral decubitus

consider administering an additional dose of epinephrine within 5–10 minutes of the first dose (while other supportive measures are being instituted as well). After failure respond to a second dose of epinephrine, it would be reasonable to consider treatment with other alternatives as below.

Intravenous Epinephrine

All current guidelines for the management of anaphylaxis suggest that intramuscular (IM) epinephrine is preferred over intravenous (IV) epinephrine [1–5]. This is due the ability to give IM dosing "in the field" by untrained personnel, the pharmacologic properties of epinephrine when given by the IM route, and the potential of the IV form to cause fatal arrhythmias and blood pressure spikes (especially if given as a bolus). However, IV epinephrine could be considered in patients with severe hypotension and/or cardiovascular collapse that fail to respond to IM epinephrine [48]. One prospective study analyzed the use of IV epinephrine (with a protocol for titration according to severity of reaction and side effects), in addition to other supportive measures, in patients with venom allergy who had systemic reactions during insect sting challenge (protocol and dosing shown in Table 3.2). This study showed a consistent and rapid resolution of anaphylaxis when intravenous epinephrine infusion was started per protocol early after onset of systemic reaction. Infusions were continued for a median duration of 115 minutes (range 52–292 minutes), and median total dose required was 590 μg (range 190–1310 μg). In some patients, the symptoms returned upon cessation of the infusion and improved after restarting the infusion, giving further evidence to the true efficacy of this therapy [49]. However, this study was conducted in a controlled setting in which patients were already

Table 3.2 Treatment guidelines

1. Oxygen	High flow oxygen by facemask if SpO_2 <92 or SBP <90 mmHg
2. Epinephrine infusion	1 mg in 100 mL (1:100,000 or 10 μg/mL) intravenously by infusion pump
	Start at 30–100 mL/hr (5–15 μg/min) according to reaction severity
	Titrate according to response and side effects, aiming for lowest effective infusion rate. Tachycardia, tremor, and pallor in the setting of a normal or raised blood pressure are signs of epinephrine toxicity; consider a reduction in infusion rate
	Stop infusion 30 minutes after resolution of all signs and symptoms
	Continue observation for at least 2 hours after ceasing infusion (longer for severe or complicated reactions)
3. Normal saline rapid infusion	1000 mL infused over 1–3 minutes and repeat as necessary
	Give if hypotension is severe or does not respond promptly to adrenaline
4. Hypotension resistant to the above measures	Consider bolus adrenaline, glucagon (5–10 mg IV bolus followed by infusion), and noradrenaline infusion with invasive blood pressure monitoring and central venous access

Adapted from Prospective Study [1]

equipped for monitoring (EKG, pulse oximetry, spirometry, and blood pressure monitoring) and treatment (IV cannula already in place, epinephrine pre-mixed and ready for IV infusion). While this was appropriate for a research setting, it is not as applicable in standard cases of anaphylaxis management (though could be considered in such settings such as planned desensitization or challenge).

Of course, adverse effects of intravenous epinephrine must be considered if this therapy is to be used. In the previously mentioned sting challenge study, the authors reported no adverse effects due to the therapy [49]. However, there are multiple case reports highlighting adverse effect of IV epinephrine [46, 50–52]. In the majority of these cases, the adverse events were associated with inappropriate dosing and bolus administration of epinephrine, rather than given as a drip or slower infusion. Thus, based on available evidence, the benefits of IV epinephrine seem to outweigh the risks if given as an infusion in refractory anaphylaxis, especially in cases where continuous hemodynamic monitoring is available, and the current guidelines do support its use for the treatment of refractory anaphylaxis [1–4, 53].

Vasopressors

Similar to IV epinephrine, there are no high-quality controlled studies on the use of vasopressors in the treatment of anaphylaxis [54]. Nevertheless, it should be considered in cases of refractory hypotension not responding to first-line agents such as epinephrine and volume resuscitation. A systemic review of vasopressors for hypotensive shock (not just limited to hypotensive shock from anaphylaxis) was unable to provide an evidence-based recommendation for any one investigated vasopressor over another [55], but consensus guidelines for anaphylaxis all support consideration of dopamine for the treatment of hypotension refractory to traditional therapies [1, 3, 4, 53]. There are other options as well however. In one study of insect sting challenge-induced anaphylaxis, there were three cases of refractory anaphylaxis. In one of these cases, norepinephrine was able to reverse hypotension, after failure of IV epinephrine to do so [56]. Finally, while not a vasopressor, atropine has been used in conjunction with IV epinephrine to combat bradycardia refractory to epinephrine [49].

Glucagon

Patients taking β-adrenergic blockers may experience refractory hypotension even after proper administration of epinephrine and other supportive measures. Glucagon has positive chronotropic effects (and possibly positive ionotropic effects) on the heart, independent of the beta-adrenergic receptor [57], and thus should always be considered in the treatment of refractory anaphylaxis in patients on β-adrenergic blockers [48]. There are limited case reports supporting its use in reversing otherwise refractory hypotension and bronchospasm from anaphylaxis [58–60]. Interestingly, the case reports that clearly show effect suggest it can stabilize blood pressure, and these were in radiocontrast-induced anaphylaxis [58, 60]. No randomized controlled trials have been performed, but there is enough agreement regarding its use that consensus guidelines recommend it [1, 3, 4, 53]. Given its potential to cause significant nausea and vomiting, one may need to consider airway protection prior to glucagon administration, especially in an obtunded patient [48].

Potential Newer Considerations for Second-Line Treatment

The previously discussed treatments are generally agreed upon as necessary or potential treatments of anaphylaxis and refractory anaphylaxis. However, in cases where anaphylaxis remains refractory to these traditional first-line or second-line agents, there are limited reports of other non-traditional agents to consider.

Methylene Blue

Methylene blue is an aromatic molecule that has been used since the late 1800s in a variety of disease states ranging from malaria to carbon monoxide poisoning [61]. Histamine and other mediators of anaphylaxis exert effects partially by inducing production of nitric oxide (NO); methylene blue is thought to exert its effects via inhibition of NO-mediated smooth muscle relaxation in the vasculature [62]. Thus, the major effects would be reversal of hypotension, without any inotropic or chronotropic effects. Methylene blue has shown to be of use in multiple case reports of distributive shock (whether from anaphylaxis or other causes) [61]. In some of these cases, the anaphylactic shock was refractory to epinephrine, norepinephrine, dopamine, and fluids and responded to methylene blue within 10–20 minutes [63–65]. Another case report suggests that it may even be beneficial in the treatment of refractory anaphylaxis without hypotension, though this is more controversial [66].

Interestingly, methylene blue has also been found to be a causative agent of anaphylaxis when used intraoperatively to identify sentinel lymph nodes or for fistula detection; however, it appears to be the safest blue dye in that regard [67]. In fact, in at least some cases of methylene blue-induced anaphylaxis, it appears that the causative agent was actually another blue dye and that methylene blue was inappropriately labeled or identified [68]. It has also been shown to cause anaphylaxis in cases of plasma transfusions treated with methylene blue, although it is often debatable how often it is the true culprit in these reactions [69]. The most recent US practice parameter mentions methylene blue in the context of causing anaphylaxis (rather than treating it), warning practitioners to consider this as a cause of perioperative anaphylaxis [3]. Regardless, if one choose to use methylene blue in the treatment of refractory anaphylaxis, some caution must be taken. Side effects include hemolytic anemia (at lower doses); nausea, vomiting, abdominal pain, fever, and hemolysis (at intermediate doses); and hypotension (at high doses). Additionally, it interferes with traditional methods of pulse oximetry and thus may cause factitious desaturations [70].

Clearly more studies on the use of methylene blue for the treatment of refractory anaphylaxis need to be conducted for it to be routinely recommended. One could consider it in certain cases of refractory anaphylaxis if appropriate monitoring parameters are in place.

Sugammadex

Sugammadex is a relatively new agent indicated for the reversal of certain paralytics. Similar to methylene blue, conflicting data exists as to whether it is a potential causative agent versus a potential adjunct treatment of perioperative anaphylaxis.

There are numerous case reports of intraoperative anaphylaxis caused by sugammadex [71], several of which have been confirmed with positive skin-prick/intradermal testing to sugammadex [72, 73]. Conversely, there are also case reports suggesting that it may be of benefit in refractory perioperative anaphylaxis caused by neuromuscular blocking agents [74, 75]. One case-control study of 13 cases of presumed rocuronium or antibiotic-induced perioperative anaphylaxis treated with sugammadex concluded that it was not beneficial [76]; however, the design and conclusion of this report have also been criticized [77]. Clearly, more research needs to be done before the use of sugammadex can be routinely recommended for refractory anaphylaxis.

Tranexamic Acid

Disseminated intravascular coagulation (DIC) has been shown to be associated with fatal anaphylaxis in up to 12% of cases [48, 78]. There is one case report of DIC-associated anaphylaxis reported to be successfully treated with tranexamic acid [79]. However, as with other questionable agents such as methylene blue and sugammadex, there are also reported cases of tranexamic acid-induced anaphylaxis [80, 81]. Clearly, this is an area where more research needs to be done in order to determine whether or not tranexamic acid is effective in the treatment of anaphylaxis.

Conclusion

Refractory anaphylaxis represents a significant percentage of cases of anaphylaxis. Risk factors are similar to those for severe anaphylaxis and include (but are not limited to) age ≥65 years, underlying cardiac/lung disease, and delayed administration of epinephrine. Experts agree that rapid treatment with IM epinephrine is the first-line treatment for diagnosis. Repeat dose(s) and/or IV epinephrine could also be considered in cases of refractory anaphylaxis. Other widely acceptable second-line agents include supine positioning, oxygen administration, and treatment with β2-agonists, H1/H2 blocking agents, corticosteroids, fluid replacement therapy and/or vasopressors, and glucagon. Other emerging and more controversial agents include methylene blue, sugammadex, and tranexamic acid, though there is not enough data for these novel treatments to be routinely recommended.

References

1. Simons FE, Ardusso LR, Bilo MB, Cardona V, Ebisawa M, El-Gamal YM, et al. International consensus on (ICON) anaphylaxis. World Allergy Organ J. 2014;7(1):9.
2. Muraro A, Roberts G, Worm M, Bilo MB, Brockow K, Fernandez Rivas M, et al. Anaphylaxis: guidelines from the European Academy of Allergy and Clinical Immunology. Allergy. 2014;69(8):1026–45.

3. Lieberman P, Nicklas RA, Randolph C, Oppenheimer J, Bernstein D, Bernstein J, et al. Anaphylaxis – a practice parameter update 2015. Ann Allergy Asthma Immunol. 2015;115(5):341–84.
4. Simons FE, Ardusso LR, Bilo MB, Dimov V, Ebisawa M, El-Gamal YM, et al. 2012 Update: World Allergy Organization Guidelines for the assessment and management of anaphylaxis. Curr Opin Allergy Clin Immunol. 2012;12(4):389–99.
5. Sampson HA, Munoz-Furlong A, Campbell RL, Adkinson NF Jr, Bock SA, Branum A, et al. Second symposium on the definition and management of anaphylaxis: summary report – Second National Institute of Allergy and Infectious Disease/Food Allergy and Anaphylaxis Network symposium. J Allergy Clin Immunol. 2006;117(2):391–7.
6. Francuzik W, Dolle S, Worm M. Risk factors and treatment of refractory anaphylaxis - a review of case reports. Expert Rev Clin Immunol. 2018;14(4):307–14.
7. Gouel-Cheron A, Harpan A, Mertes PM, Longrois D. Management of anaphylactic shock in the operating room. Presse Med. 2016;45(9):774–83.
8. Tejedor Alonso MA, Moro Moro M, Mugica Garcia MV. Epidemiology of anaphylaxis. Clin Exp Allergy. 2015;45(6):1027–39.
9. Mullins RJ, Wainstein BK, Barnes EH, Liew WK, Campbell DE. Increases in anaphylaxis fatalities in Australia from 1997 to 2013. Clin Exp Allergy. 2016;46(8):1099–110.
10. Sclar DA, Lieberman PL. Anaphylaxis: underdiagnosed, underreported, and undertreated. Am J Med. 2014;127(1 Suppl):S1–5.
11. Motosue MS, Bellolio MF, Van Houten HK, Shah ND, Campbell RL. Risk factors for severe anaphylaxis in the United States. Ann Allergy Asthma Immunol. 2017;119(4):356–61. e2
12. Clark S, Wei W, Rudders SA, Camargo CA Jr. Risk factors for severe anaphylaxis in patients receiving anaphylaxis treatment in US emergency departments and hospitals. J Allergy Clin Immunol. 2014;134(5):1125–30.
13. Bock SA, Munoz-Furlong A, Sampson HA. Fatalities due to anaphylactic reactions to foods. J Allergy Clin Immunol. 2001;107(1):191–3.
14. Sampson HA, Mendelson L, Rosen JP. Fatal and near-fatal anaphylactic reactions to food in children and adolescents. N Engl J Med. 1992;327(6):380–4.
15. Yunginger JW, Sweeney KG, Sturner WQ, Giannandrea LA, Teigland JD, Bray M, et al. Fatal food-induced anaphylaxis. JAMA. 1988;260(10):1450–2.
16. Pumphrey RS, Gowland MH. Further fatal allergic reactions to food in the United Kingdom, 1999-2006. J Allergy Clin Immunol. 2007;119(4):1018–9.
17. Grabenhenrich L, Hompes S, Gough H, Rueff F, Scherer K, Pfohler C, et al. Implementation of anaphylaxis management guidelines: a register-based study. PLoS One. 2012;7(5):e35778.
18. Turner PJ, Jerschow E, Umasunthar T, Lin R, Campbell DE, Boyle RJ. Fatal anaphylaxis: mortality rate and risk factors. J Allergy Clin Immunol Pract. 2017;5(5):1169–78.
19. Simons KJ, Simons FE. Epinephrine and its use in anaphylaxis: current issues. Curr Opin Allergy Clin Immunol. 2010;10(4):354–61.
20. Fineman SM, Bowman SH, Campbell RL, Dowling P, O'Rourke D, Russell WS, et al. Addressing barriers to emergency anaphylaxis care: from emergency medical services to emergency department to outpatient follow-up. Ann Allergy Asthma Immunol. 2015;115(4):301–5.
21. Stewart WJ, McSweeney SM, Kellett MA, Faxon DP, Ryan TJ. Increased risk of severe protamine reactions in NPH insulin-dependent diabetics undergoing cardiac catheterization. Circulation. 1984;70(5):788–92.
22. Dewachter P, Mouton-Faivre C, Hepner DL. Perioperative anaphylaxis: what should be known? Curr Allergy Asthma Rep. 2015;15(5):21.
23. Lieberman JA, Chehade M. Use of omalizumab in the treatment of food allergy and anaphylaxis. Curr Allergy Asthma Rep. 2013;13(1):78–84.
24. Warrier P, Casale TB. Omalizumab in idiopathic anaphylaxis. Ann Allergy Asthma Immunol. 2009;102(3):257–8.
25. Pitt TJ, Cisneros N, Kalicinsky C, Becker AB. Successful treatment of idiopathic anaphylaxis in an adolescent. J Allergy Clin Immunol. 2010;126(2):415–6. author reply 6

26. Jones JD, Marney SR Jr, Fahrenholz JM. Idiopathic anaphylaxis successfully treated with omalizumab. Ann Allergy Asthma Immunol. 2008;101(5):550–1.
27. Demirturk M, Gelincik A, Colakoglu B, Dal M, Buyukozturk S. Promising option in the prevention of idiopathic anaphylaxis: omalizumab. J Dermatol. 2012;39(6):552–4.
28. Bell MC, Jackson DJ. Prevention of anaphylaxis related to mast cell activation syndrome with omalizumab. Ann Allergy Asthma Immunol. 2012;108(5):383–4.
29. Carter MC, Robyn JA, Bressler PB, Walker JC, Shapiro GG, Metcalfe DD. Omalizumab for the treatment of unprovoked anaphylaxis in patients with systemic mastocytosis. J Allergy Clin Immunol. 2007;119(6):1550–1.
30. Douglass JA, Carroll K, Voskamp A, Bourke P, Wei A, O'Hehir RE. Omalizumab is effective in treating systemic mastocytosis in a nonatopic patient. Allergy. 2010;65(7):926–7.
31. Kontou-Fili K, Filis CI, Voulgari C, Panayiotidis PG. Omalizumab monotherapy for bee sting and unprovoked "anaphylaxis" in a patient with systemic mastocytosis and undetectable specific IgE. Ann Allergy Asthma Immunol. 2010;104(6):537–9.
32. Molderings GJ, Raithel M, Kratz F, Azemar M, Haenisch B, Harzer S, et al. Omalizumab treatment of systemic mast cell activation disease: experiences from four cases. Intern Med. 2011;50(6):611–5.
33. Jagdis A, Vadas P. Omalizumab effectively prevents recurrent refractory anaphylaxis in a patient with monoclonal mast cell activation syndrome. Ann Allergy Asthma Immunol. 2014;113(1):115–6.
34. Choo KJ, Simons FE, Sheikh A. Glucocorticoids for the treatment of anaphylaxis. Cochrane Database Syst Rev. 2012;(4):CD007596.
35. Sheikh A. Glucocorticosteroids for the treatment and prevention of anaphylaxis. Curr Opin Allergy Clin Immunol. 2013;13(3):263–7.
36. Alqurashi W, Ellis AK. Do corticosteroids prevent biphasic anaphylaxis? J Allergy Clin Immunol Pract. 2017;5(5):1194–205.
37. Brown AF, McKinnon D, Chu K. Emergency department anaphylaxis: a review of 142 patients in a single year. J Allergy Clin Immunol. 2001;108(5):861–6.
38. Gaeta TJ, Clark S, Pelletier AJ, Camargo CA. National study of US emergency department visits for acute allergic reactions, 1993 to 2004. Ann Allergy Asthma Immunol. 2007;98(4):360–5.
39. Worm M, Moneret-Vautrin A, Scherer K, Lang R, Fernandez-Rivas M, Cardona V, et al. First European data from the network of severe allergic reactions (NORA). Allergy. 2014;69(10):1397–404.
40. Lieberman P, Nicklas RA, Oppenheimer J, Kemp SF, Lang DM, Bernstein DI, et al. The diagnosis and management of anaphylaxis practice parameter: 2010 update. J Allergy Clin Immunol. 2010;126(3):477–80. e1–42.
41. Kemp AM, Kemp SF. Pharmacotherapy in refractory anaphylaxis: when intramuscular epinephrine fails. Curr Opin Allergy Clin Immunol. 2014;14(4):371–8.
42. Pumphrey RS. Lessons for management of anaphylaxis from a study of fatal reactions. Clin Exp Allergy. 2000;30(8):1144–50.
43. Macdougall CF, Cant AJ, Colver AF. How dangerous is food allergy in childhood? The incidence of severe and fatal allergic reactions across the UK and Ireland. Arch Dis Child. 2002;86(4):236–9.
44. Brown JC. Epinephrine, auto-injectors, and anaphylaxis: challenges of dose, depth, and device. Ann Allergy Asthma Immunol. 2018;121(1):53–60.
45. Simons FE, Edwards ES, Read EJ Jr, Clark S, Liebelt EL. Voluntarily reported unintentional injections from epinephrine auto-injectors. J Allergy Clin Immunol. 2010;125(2):419–23. e4
46. Wood JP, Traub SJ, Lipinski C. Safety of epinephrine for anaphylaxis in the emergency setting. World J Emerg Med. 2013;4(4):245–51.
47. Edwards ES, Gunn R, Simons ER, Carr K, Chinchilli VM, Painter G, et al. Bioavailability of epinephrine from Auvi-Q compared with EpiPen. Ann Allergy Asthma Immunol. 2013;111(2):132–7.
48. Brown SGAKS, Lieberman PL. Anaphylaxis. In: Adkinson Jr NFBB, Burks AW, et al., editors. Middleton's allergy: principles and practice. 2. 8th ed. Philadelphia: Elsevier Saunders; 2014. p. 1237–59.

49. Brown SG, Blackman KE, Stenlake V, Heddle RJ. Insect sting anaphylaxis; prospective evaluation of treatment with intravenous adrenaline and volume resuscitation. Emerg Med J. 2004;21(2):149–54.
50. Campbell RL, Bellolio MF, Knutson BD, Bellamkonda VR, Fedko MG, Nestler DM, et al. Epinephrine in anaphylaxis: higher risk of cardiovascular complications and overdose after administration of intravenous bolus epinephrine compared with intramuscular epinephrine. J Allergy Clin Immunol Pract. 2015;3(1):76–80.
51. Kanwar M, Irvin CB, Frank JJ, Weber K, Rosman H. Confusion about epinephrine dosing leading to iatrogenic overdose: a life-threatening problem with a potential solution. Ann Emerg Med. 2010;55(4):341–4.
52. Khoueiry G, Abi Rafeh N, Azab B, Markman E, Waked A, AbouRjaili G, et al. Reverse Takotsubo cardiomyopathy in the setting of anaphylaxis treated with high-dose intravenous epinephrine. J Emerg Med. 2013;44(1):96–9.
53. Soar J, Perkins GD, Abbas G, Alfonzo A, Barelli A, Bierens JJ, et al. European Resuscitation Council Guidelines for Resuscitation 2010 Section 8. Cardiac arrest in special circumstances: electrolyte abnormalities, poisoning, drowning, accidental hypothermia, hyperthermia, asthma, anaphylaxis, cardiac surgery, trauma, pregnancy, electrocution. Resuscitation. 2010;81(10):1400–33.
54. Dhami S, Panesar SS, Roberts G, Muraro A, Worm M, Bilo MB, et al. Management of anaphylaxis: a systematic review. Allergy. 2014;69(2):168–75.
55. Havel C, Arrich J, Losert H, Gamper G, Mullner M, Herkner H. Vasopressors for hypotensive shock. Cochrane Database Syst Rev. 2011;(5):CD003709.
56. Smith PL, Kagey-Sobotka A, Bleecker ER, Traystman R, Kaplan AP, Gralnick H, et al. Physiologic manifestations of human anaphylaxis. J Clin Invest. 1980;66(5):1072–80.
57. Hernandez-Cascales J. Does glucagon have a positive inotropic effect in the human heart? Cardiovasc Diabetol. 2018;17(1):148.
58. Javeed N, Javeed H, Javeed S, Moussa G, Wong P, Rezai F. Refractory anaphylactoid shock potentiated by beta-blockers. Catheter Cardiovasc Diagn. 1996;39(4):383–4.
59. Thomas M, Crawford I. Best evidence topic report. Glucagon infusion in refractory anaphylactic shock in patients on beta-blockers. Emerg Med J. 2005;22(4):272–3.
60. Zaloga GP, DeLacey W, Holmboe E, Chernow B. Glucagon reversal of hypotension in a case of anaphylactoid shock. Ann Intern Med. 1986;105(1):65–6.
61. Jang DH, Nelson LS, Hoffman RS. Methylene blue for distributive shock: a potential new use of an old antidote. J Med Toxicol. 2013;9(3):242–9.
62. Evora PR, Simon MR. Role of nitric oxide production in anaphylaxis and its relevance for the treatment of anaphylactic hypotension with methylene blue. Ann Allergy Asthma Immunol. 2007;99(4):306–13.
63. Da Silva PS, Furtado P. Methylene blue to treat refractory latex-induced anaphylactic shock: a case report. A A Pract. 2018;10(3):57–60.
64. Del Duca D, Sheth SS, Clarke AE, Lachapelle KJ, Ergina PL. Use of methylene blue for catecholamine-refractory vasoplegia from protamine and aprotinin. Ann Thorac Surg. 2009;87(2):640–2.
65. Oliveira Neto AM, Duarte NM, Vicente WV, Viaro F, Evora PR. Methylene blue: an effective treatment for contrast medium-induced anaphylaxis. Med Sci Monit. 2003;9(11):CS102–6.
66. Bauer CS, Vadas P, Kelly KJ. Methylene blue for the treatment of refractory anaphylaxis without hypotension. Am J Emerg Med. 2013;31(1):264 e3–5.
67. Ramin S, Azar FP, Malihe H. Methylene blue as the safest blue dye for sentinel node mapping: emphasis on anaphylaxis reaction. Acta Oncol. 2011;50(5):729–31.
68. Li PH, Wagner A, York M, Rutkowski R, Haque R, Rutkowski K. Blue dye allergy: pitfalls in diagnosis and how to avoid them. J Allergy Clin Immunol Pract. 2018;6(1):272–3.
69. Mertes PM, Demoly P, Alperovitch A, Bazin A, Bienvenu J, Caldani C, et al. Methylene blue-treated plasma: an increased allergy risk? J Allergy Clin Immunol. 2012;130(3):808–12.
70. Clifton J 2nd, Leikin JB. Methylene blue. Am J Ther. 2003;10(4):289–91.
71. Takazawa T, Mitsuhata H, Mertes PM. Sugammadex and rocuronium-induced anaphylaxis. J Anesth. 2016;30(2):290–7.

72. Ue KL, Kasternow B, Wagner A, Rutkowski R, Rutkowski K. Sugammadex: an emerging trigger of intraoperative anaphylaxis. Ann Allergy Asthma Immunol. 2016;117(6):714–6.
73. Nakanishi T, Ishida K, Utada K, Yamaguchi M, Matsumoto M. Anaphylaxis to sugammadex diagnosed by skin prick testing using both sugammadex and a sugammadex-rocuronium mixture. Anaesth Intensive Care. 2016;44(1):122–4.
74. Barthel F, Stojeba N, Lyons G, Biermann C, Diemunsch P. Sugammadex in rocuronium anaphylaxis: dose matters. Br J Anaesth. 2012;109(4):646–7.
75. McDonnell NJ, Pavy TJ, Green LK, Platt PR. Sugammadex in the management of rocuronium-induced anaphylaxis. Br J Anaesth. 2011;106(2):199–201.
76. Platt PR, Clarke RC, Johnson GH, Sadleir PH. Efficacy of sugammadex in rocuronium-induced or antibiotic-induced anaphylaxis. A case-control study. Anaesthesia. 2015;70(11):1264–7.
77. Whitehead A. Sugammadex in anaphylaxis. A case-control study? Anaesthesia. 2016;71(2):236–7.
78. Pumphrey R. Anaphylaxis: can we tell who is at risk of a fatal reaction? Curr Opin Allergy Clin Immunol. 2004;4(4):285–90.
79. De Souza RL, Short T, Warman GR, Maclennan N, Young Y. Anaphylaxis with associated fibrinolysis, reversed with tranexamic acid and demonstrated by thrombelastography. Anaesth Intensive Care. 2004;32(4):580–7.
80. Bansal RA, Nicholas A, Bansal AS. Tranexamic acid: an exceedingly rare cause of anaphylaxis during anaesthesia. Case Rep Immunol. 2016;2016:7828351.
81. Li PH, Trigg C, Rutkowski R, Rutkowski K. Anaphylaxis to tranexamic acid-a rare reaction to a common drug. J Allergy Clin Immunol Pract. 2017;5(3):839–41.

Biphasic Anaphylaxis: Epidemiology, Predictors, and Management

4

Waleed Alqurashi

Introduction

Anaphylaxis is the most severe form of allergy that rapidly affects multiple body systems and can be deadly [1, 2]. Most anaphylactic reactions are uniphasic, with early allergic responses that occur minutes after exposure and typically subside with time without recurring. However, some have biphasic responses. Biphasic anaphylaxis (BA) is the recurrence of anaphylactic symptoms after initial resolution, despite no further exposure to the trigger [3–5]. Studies in the 1980s and 1990s showed that BA could be fatal or near-fatal [6]. Although reports of fatal biphasic reactions are rare in recent literature, severe late reactions that require advanced airway intervention, extracorporeal membrane oxygenation resuscitation, and intensive care monitoring continue to be reported [7–10].

Epidemiology of Biphasic Anaphylaxis

Table 4.1 provides an up-to-date summary of the studies that reported the incidence of biphasic reactions regardless of the nature or severity of the secondary reaction. Interestingly, the reported incidence of this potentially life-threatening phenomenon varies from 3% to 23%, with most occurring 1–24 h from the onset of the initial reaction. However, some studies reported recurrence up to 72 h, particularly among adult patients [7, 11]. This wide range in the reported incidence is due to several epidemiological factors. Overall, the published studies to date vary considerably in their design, enrolled population (adults vs children or mixed), settings (emergency rooms vs outpatient clinics), and definition and severity of anaphylaxis and biphasic

W. Alqurashi (✉)

Division of Emergency Medicine, Department of Pediatrics,
University of Ottawa, Children's Hospital of Eastern Ontario, Ottawa, ON, Canada
e-mail: walqurashi@cheo.on.ca

© Springer Nature Switzerland AG 2020

A. K. Ellis (ed.), *Anaphylaxis*, https://doi.org/10.1007/978-3-030-43205-8_4

Table 4.1 Summary of previous studies on biphasic anaphylaxis

Study/year	Design	Settings and subjects	Incidence (%)	Nature	Age (y)	Trigger	Time to onset (h)[a]	Risk factors	Association with corticosteroids
Popa and Lerner [21], 1984	Case series	Adults three cases (all M[b])	NR[b]	A[b]	22–52	1 immunotherapy 1 insect bite 1 rabies vaccine in patient with egg allergy	3–4	NR	(2 patients received steroids for the initial reaction) Route, IV[b] Time, NR
Stark and Sullivan [6], 1986	Prospective	Adults inpatients and ED[b] 5/25 developed BR[b] (3 F[b], 2 M)	20%	A	21–67	4 drugs (antibiotics) 1 radiocontrast media	1–8	Anaphylaxis provoked by oral trigger. Delay of ≥30 min between exposure to trigger and development of initial reaction. Severe initial symptoms not predictive of BR	NAI Route, IV Time, within 1 h of arrival to ED
Sampson et al. [76], 1992	Case series	13 Children three developed fatal BR (2 F, 1 M)	23%	A	8–15	Food (1 peanut, 2 tree nuts)	1–2	All patients with BR had asthma. Delay in administration of first epinephrine after ingestion of allergen for all three patients	NR
Douglas et al. [11], 1994	Retrospective	Adults ED, inpatients, and outpatient allergy clinic 4/59 had BR (1 F, 3 M)	7%	2 A 2 NA[b]	20–77	2 drugs 2 food (shrimp)	Mean 30 (range 1–72)	No clinical features distinguished patients with UR from BR. However, 50% of patients with BR had hypotension that required treatment with IV fluids compared to 16% of those with UR[b]	NAI Route and time, NR
Brady et al. [77], 1997	Retrospective	Adults ED visits 2/67 developed BR (1 F, 1 M)	3%	NA	19–21	Hymenoptera envenomation	Mean 33 (range 26–40)	None	NAI Route, IV/PO[b] Time, NR

Brazil and MacNamara [40], 1998	Retrospective	Adults ED visits 6/34 developed BR	18%	A	NR	3 insect bites 1 food (nuts) 2 drugs	Mean 16.3 (range 4.5–29.5)	Patients with BR required larger doses of epinephrine to treat their initial reaction	NR
Lee and Greenes [54], 2000	Retrospective	Children hospital admissions 6/105 developed BR (3 F, 3 M)	6%	3 A 3 NA	1–13	2 drugs 2 food (fish, nuts) 2 bee stings	Mean 10.1 (range 1.3–28.4)	Delay in epinephrine administration	NAI Route and time, NR
Smit et al. [78], 2005	Retrospective	Adults and children ED visits 15/282 developed BR (5 F, 10 M)	5.3%	3 A 12 NA	6–80	5 food (seafood) 4 drugs 5 unknown 1 insect bite	Mean 8 (range 1.4–23)	Delay in presentation to ED (1 h for UR vs 3 h for BR) 20% of patients with BR had unstable vital signs on initial presentation to ED	NAI Route, IV Mean time to treatment 7.57 h (SD 5.46)
Poachanukoon and Paopairochanakorn [57], 2006	Retrospective	Adults and children hospital admissions 8/52 developed BR (4 F, 4 M)	15%	NR	NR	NR	NR	Time interval between the onset of initial reaction and the first epinephrine was longer for patients with BR	NAI Route and time, NR
Jirapongsananuruk et al. [79], 2007	Retrospective	Hospitalized mixed population 5/101 developed BR	5%	NR	NR	NR	NR	NR	NAI Route and time, NR
Ellis and Day [58], 2007	Prospective	Adults and children ED visits and hospital admissions 20/103 developed BR (9 F, 11 M)	19.4%	A	4–73	7 unknown 5 hymenoptera 6 food 1 drug 1 immunotherapy	Mean 10 (range 1.5–38)	Patients with BR received less total epinephrine dose and less systemic steroid treatment for their initial reactions	Biphasic reactors received less corticosteroid (P = 0.06) Route and time, NR

(continued)

Table 4.1 (continued)

Study/year	Design	Settings and subjects	Incidence (%)	Nature	Age (y)	Trigger	Time to onset (h)[a]	Risk factors	Association with corticosteroids
Scranton et al. [41], 2009	Prospective	Adults and children allergy clinic 14/60 developed BR (13 F, 1 M)	23%	NA	25–66	Immunotherapy	Mean 7.2 (range 2–24)	Patients in the BR group were more likely to require multiple epinephrine treatments for the initial reaction	NAI Route, oral Time, NR
Mehr et al. [42], 2009	Retrospective	Children ED visits 12/109 developed BR (4 F, 8 M)	11%	5 A 7 NA	0.2–17	9 food 2 unknown 1 drug	Mean 9.5 (range 1.2–20.5)	Children who received >1 dose of epinephrine and/ or a fluid bolus treatment of their initial anaphylactic reaction were at increased risk of BR	NAI Route, PO/IV Median time to administration, 108 min (IQR 20–260)
Confino-Cohen et al. [80], 2010	Prospective	Adults and children allergy clinic 10/112 developed BR (7 F, 3 M)	9%	NA	14–48	Immunotherapy	3–24	Relatively low peak expiratory flow (PEF) (regardless of asthma history) at baseline and concomitant asthma are possible risk factors for BR	NR
Lertnawapan and Maekanantawat [55], 2011	Retrospective	Adult and PED ED visits 13/208 developed BR (9 F, 4 M)	6.3%	A	Median 18	4 seafood 2 fried insect as food 2 immunotherapy 1 insecticide 4 unknown	Mean 8 (range 2–13)	Median time from the onset of the initial reaction to hospital arrival and to 1st epinephrine treatment was significantly longer in patient with BR compared to those with UR	NAI Route and time, NR
Orhan et al. [81], 2011	Retrospective	PED clinic 7/224 developed BR	3.1%	A	Median 3	3 food 2 drugs 1 immunotherapy 1 hymenoptera	1.5–6	NR	NR

Inoue et al. [43], 2013	Retrospective	Children inpatient and outpatient visits 2/61 developed BR (1 F, 1 M)	3.3%	A	4–7.5	NR	12–18	Patients who developed BR were more likely to have experienced syncope, vomiting, and treatment with >1 dose of epinephrine for their initial reactions	NAI Route, IV/PO Time, NR
Lee et al. [82], 2013	Retrospective	Pediatric allergy clinic 9/614 developed BR (4 F, 5 M)	1.5%	4 A 5 NA	0.2–17	Oral food challenge to milk, egg, and peanut	2–24	Patients with BPR were significantly more likely to have received steroids for their initial reaction. BR seem to be associated with the severity of the initial reaction	NAI Route, PO Time, NR
Nagano et al. [83], 2013	Retrospective	PED ED 3/340 developed BR	<1%	A	Median 3	NR	3–28	NR	NAI Route, IV/PO Time, NR
Vezir et al. [84], 2013	Prospective	Pediatric allergy clinic 5/96 developed BR (3 F, 2 M)	5.2%	NR	<5y = 1 >5y = 4	3 drugs 2 hymenoptera	0.5–9	All patients with BR had received fluid therapy for their initial reaction, which was severe in four of them	NAI Route and time, NR
Liew et al. [85], 2013	Retrospective	PEDs ED/allergy clinic 4/108 developed BR	3.7%	NR	NR	NR	All within 24	Three patients required intensive care unit stay for hypotension at presentation	NR
Brown et al. [17], 2013	Prospective	Adult ED 55/412 developed BR	13%	29 A (treated with epinephrine)	NR	NR	0.2–30.4	Pre-existing lung disease and initially severe reactions (hypotension)	NAI Route and time, NR
Grunau et al. [74], 2014	Retrospective	Adult ED, 2/496 developed BR (2 M)	0.4%	NA	37–38	1 food 1 drug	0.26–3.3	None identified	NAI Route, IV Time, NR

(continued)

Table 4.1 (continued)

Study/year	Design	Settings and subjects	Incidence (%)	Nature	Age (y)	Trigger	Time to onset (h)[a]	Risk factors	Association with corticosteroids
Rohacek et al. [86], 2014	Retrospective	Adult ED, 25/532 developed BR (19 F, 6 M)	4.7%	12 A 13 NA	Mean 42.3 (SD 15.2	9 food 6 drugs 3 hymenoptera 7 unknown	12 (1–36)	None identified	NAI (in subset of patients with initial anaphylactic reaction) Route and time, NR
Lee et al. [7], 2014	Retrospective	Adult ED, 21/541 developed BR (13 F, 8 M)	3.9%	A	Median 41 (IQR 31–51)	4 food 5 drugs 1 hymenoptera 9 Unknown 2 Other	Median 7 (range 1–72)	Prior anaphylaxis, unknown trigger, wheezing, and diarrhea	NAI Route and time, NR
Oya et al. [87], 2014	Retrospective	Hospitalized patients from adults' ED.7/114 developed BR (4F, 3 M)	6.1%	3A 4 NA	Mean 31 (SD 27.5)	3 foods 3 drugs 1 hymenoptera	Median 8	NR	NAI Route and time, NR
Sricharoen et al. [88], 2014	Prospective	Adult ED, 10/47 developed BR (7 F, 3 M)	21.3%	9 NA 1 A	Mean 38 (SD 11.57)	4 foods 4 drugs 2 insect	Median 21.7 (range, 4.5–47)	Initial symptoms of abdominal pain Lower risk in patient with lower respiratory rate	NAI Route, NR Median time (min) 2.17 (0.67–15.75)
Manuyakorn et al. [56], 2015	Retrospective	Hospitalized children, 15/172 developed BR (5 F, 10 M)	8.7%	NR	Mean 6.5 (SD 4.6)	2 foods 10 drugs 3 blood products	NR	Patients with BR tended to be younger than those with UR, have more severe initial reaction, and are less likely to be treated with epinephrine. Lower risk of BR in patient with anaphylaxis to known previous triggers	NAI Route and time, NR

Alqurashi et al. [12], 2015	Retrospective	Pediatric ED, 71/484 developed BR (20 F, 51 M)	14.7%	49 A	Median 6 (2.7–10.1)	47 foods 3 drugs 1 bee sting 1 exercise 15 unspecified	Before ED discharge, 4.7 (3.3–6) After ED discharge, 18.5 (9.2–25.2)	Age 6–9 years, delay in presentation to ED or epinephrine administration for >90 min from the onset of the initial reaction, wide pulse pressure at triage, treatment of initial reaction with >1 dose of epinephrine, administration of inhaled β-agonists in ED	NAI Route, IV/PO Median time (min) to first dose 120 (IQR 87–256)
Ko et al. [8], 2015	Retrospective	Adult ED 9/415 developed BR (7 F, 2 M)	2.2%	A	Median 41 (range 24–60)	4 foods 5 drugs	15 (range 1–45) from resolution of initial symptoms	History of anaphylaxis to drugs	NR (only anaphylaxis patients treated with steroids were included in the study)
Saleh-Langenberg et al. [38], 2016	Retrospective	Pediatric allergy clinic 171/1142 developed both immediate and BR[c]	14.9%	67 A (moderate to severe index severity score)	Mean 5.7 (SD 4.2)	Oral food challenge to milk, egg, peanut, cashew, and hazelnut	Mean 3.5 (SD 7.6)	BR are associated with severe initial reactions after the challenge	Nr
Lee et al. [53], 2017	Mixed	Adult ED, 65/872 developed BR (23 F, 13 M)	7.5%	36 A 29 NA	Median 34 (IQR 17–53)	19 drugs 12 drugs 3 venom 4 contrast/latex 27 unknown	Median 3 (range 0.5–44) for anaphylactic BR	History of anaphylaxis, unknown inciting trigger, and delay in epinephrine administration>60 min from the onset of symptom. Dyspnea and delay in ED presentation for >90 min are associated with NA responses	NAI

(continued)

Table 4.1 (continued)

Study/year	Design	Settings and subjects	Incidence (%)	Nature	Age (y)	Trigger	Time to onset (h)[a]	Risk factors	Association with corticosteroids
Kim et al. [39], 2017	Retrospective	Radiology department of tertiary care center, 15/145 developed BR (8 F, 7 M)	10.3%	A (100% with initial cardiovascular symptoms)	Median 49 (IQR 23–75)	Iodinated contrast media	Median 4.8 (range 1.1–20.3)	Severe initial reactions (symptoms for ≥40 min before resolution, requiring continuous epinephrine infusion and intensive care admission), patients with history of allergic diseases	NAI Route, IV Median time (min) to first dose 23 (IQR 14–25)
Dribin et al. [89], 2019	Retrospective	Pediatric ED Of the 665 hospitalized from ED, 108 (16.2%) needed further inpatient therapy	NR	NR	<3y = 211 >3y = 454	389 foods 42 medications 8 venom 219 unknown	NR	Children with no wheezing, hypotension, or wide pulse pressure on initial presentation were at low risk of receipt of acute inpatient therapies during hospitalization	NR

[a]Time from the onset of the initial anaphylactic reaction to biphasic reaction

[b]Abbreviations: *NR* not reported, *A* anaphylactic, *NA* non-anaphylactic, *ED* emergency department, *F* female, *M* male, *BR* biphasic reaction, *UR* uniphasic reaction, *NAI* no association identified, *IV* intravenous, *PO* oral

[c]A total of 400 of 1141 developed late reaction: 53 (4.6%) reported late reactions both on the active challenge day and on the placebo challenge day, 237 (20.8%) only reported late reactions on the active challenge day, and 110 children (9.6%) only reported late reactions on the placebo challenge day. Only data of the active challenge day group were reported above

reaction [12–14]. These are critical factors that significantly influence the reported magnitude of the risk [14, 15]. For example, the three prospective adult emergency department (ED) studies to date reported an average BA incidence of 18.4% compared to <5.6% reported in eleven adult ED retrospective studies [5]. The significant clinical and statistical heterogeneity between previous observational studies is also underlined in a 2014 meta-analysis [13].

Settings of previous studies likely contribute to variability in reported BA incidence. Studies that enrolled ED or hospitalized patients reported a higher proportion of BA compared to patients from allergy clinics. This likely speaks to the severity of the initial anaphylactic reactions and the likely variability in the nature and severity of BA. For example, approximately 15% of children who presented to the ED with anaphylaxis developed BA [13], compared to 1.5% in children who experienced mild allergic reaction during controlled oral food challenge in an allergy clinic [16]. With all these factors in mind, the true incidence of biphasic reaction likely lies between 10% and 20% [14, 17].

Pathophysiology

Experts now believe anaphylaxis to be a syndrome in which different phenotypes and/or endotypes may be linked to the activation of various cells and immune mediators, ultimately leading to a wide variety of clinical manifestations [16]. As we currently understand it, three key types of factors influence the anaphylaxis phenotype: allergen, patient, and disease-modifying factors. These factors, in turn, affect BA risk (Fig. 4.1). Two key BA predictors, identified consistently by multiple studies, are the severity of initial anaphylaxis phase and early epinephrine therapy [5]. The strong association between anaphylaxis severity and risk of BA suggests that most BA represent a protracted inflammatory process intrinsically linked with initial reaction severity [17, 18].

Animal and human studies implicate a broad range of anaphylaxis mediators. However, relationships between mediators and their associations with reaction severity or subsequent BA have not been fully outlined. In a prospective study in adults, Stone et al. analyzed peak concentrations of mediators: histamine, tryptase, cytokines (IL-2, IL-4, IL-5, IL-6, IL-10, IL-13, interferon gamma, TNF alpha [tumor necrosis factor alpha], TNFRI [tumor necrosis factor receptor I]), and chemokines [19]. All mediators were higher in anaphylactic patients than controls. More recently, Brown et al. found that tryptase, histamine, IL-6, IL-10, and TFNRI are associated with anaphylaxis severity and subsequent development of BA [20]. This mechanism is supported by earlier studies that suggested that BA is a result of influx of inflammatory cells [21] or a second wave of mast cell degranulation [22].

Studies investigating the role of platelet-activating factor (PAF) in human anaphylaxis have indicated that serum PAF levels are significantly increased and correlate directly with the severity of anaphylaxis [17, 23]. Data reveal that PAF is a highly injurious and potentially lethal mediator of anaphylaxis [24]. The only therapies that have been shown to counter the effect of PAF are epinephrine or a

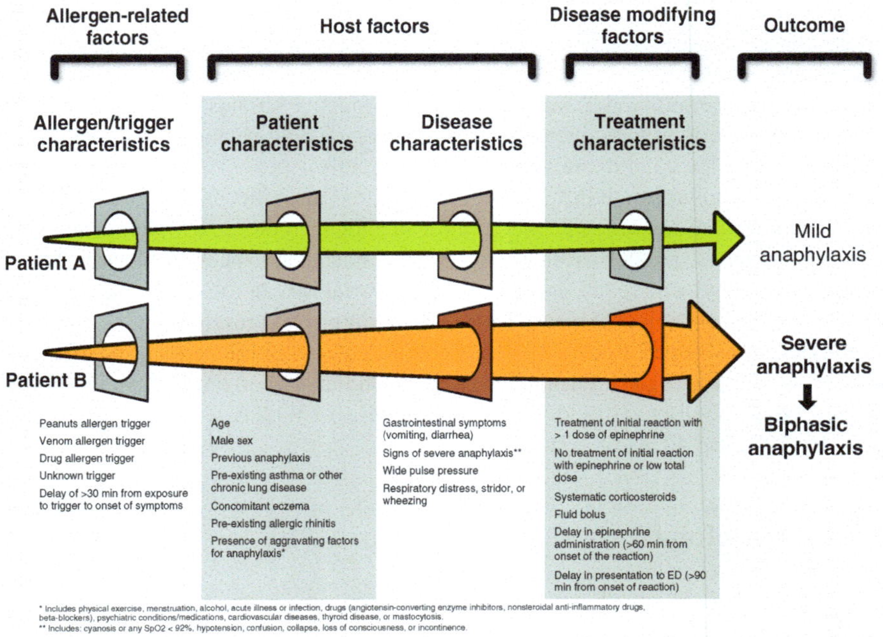
Allergen-related factors
Host factors
Disease modifying factors
Outcome
Allergen/trigger characteristics
Patient characteristics
Disease characteristics
Treatment characteristics
Patient A
Mild anaphylaxis
Patient B
Severe anaphylaxis
Biphasic anaphylaxis
Peanuts allergen trigger
Venom allergen trigger
Drug allergen trigger
Unknown trigger
Delay of >30 min from exposure to trigger to onset of symptoms
Age
Male sex
Previous anaphylaxis
Pre-existing asthma or other chronic lung disease
Concomitant eczema
Pre-existing allergic rhinitis
Presence of aggravating factors for anaphylaxis*
Gastrointestinal symptoms (vomiting, diarrhea)
Signs of severe anaphylaxis**
Wide pulse pressure
Respiratory distress, stridor, or wheezing
Treatment of initial reaction with > 1 dose of epinephrine
No treatment of initial reaction with epinephrine or low total dose
Systematic corticosteroids
Fluid bolus
Delay in epinephrine administration (>60 min from onset of the reaction)
Delay in presentation to ED (>90 min from onset of reaction)
* Includes physical exercise, menstruation, alcohol, acute illness or infection, drugs (angiotensin-converting enzyme inhibitors, nonsteroidal anti-inflammatory drugs, beta-blockers), psychiatric conditions/medications, cardiovascular diseases, thyroid disease, or mastocytosis.
** Includes: cyanosis or any SpO2 < 92%, hypotension, confusion, collapse, loss of consciousness, or incontinence.

Fig. 4.1 Clinical predictors of biphasic anaphylaxis

combination of epinephrine with methylene blue [25]. This mediator peaks within 60 to 90 minutes from the onset of anaphylaxis [26]. Vadas and Perelman examined the effect of the timing of epinephrine addition on the action of PAF and found that epinephrine was most effective when administered before stimulation with PAF but was progressively less effective with time after PAF stimulation [27]. Therefore, early administration of epinephrine is most effective in slowing or stopping the progression of anaphylaxis, whereas delayed administration of epinephrine neither interferes with PAF signalling nor favorably alters the natural history of anaphylaxis [24]. Although a study in animal found that late synthesis of PAF occurs in response to cytokines and chemotactic factors released during the initial reaction [28], human data do not support this proposed mechanism [17].

Clinical Predictors

In a recent systematic review [29], we identified potential predictors of BA. We summarized literature findings from the preceding 33 years in a conceptual model that integrates all identified potentially protective and risk factors for BA (Fig. 4.1). Given the direct association between initially severe anaphylaxis and subsequent BA, these predictors encompass all recently identified risk factors for severe anaphylaxis from the European Anaphylaxis Registry [30]. We also included potential aggravating factors for severe anaphylaxis, such as menses, co-existing infection, and drugs [31–34]. As we discussed above, the most important prognostic factors of BA, recognized consistently by multiple studies, are the severity of initial anaphylaxis phase and early epinephrine therapy [5].

Association with disease severity The best data about anaphylaxis pathophysiology is driven from near-fatal cases, especially those recorded under monitored experimental settings. These studies consistently showed that respiratory and cardiovascular manifestations are the most common indicators of severe anaphylaxis [35–37]. However, due to the lack of a valid anaphylaxis severity scoring, the definition of severity in the existing literature is inconsistent. Since most of the evidence comes from retrospective record reviews where key clinical parameters are sometimes poorly documented, an alternative strategy to examine disease severity is therapies required to reverse derangement in the cardiovascular and respiratory systems such as multiple epinephrine therapy, fluid resuscitation, or inhaled β-agonist. To date, one of the most robust reports demonstrating a "dose-response" effect of disease severity on the risk of BA was published by Brown et al. [17]. In their prospective cohort study of adults with anaphylaxis, BA was associated with increasing severity of the initial reaction (Table 4.1). Also, among children who underwent double-blind, placebo-controlled food challenge, the risk of late reactions was significantly higher in those with severe initial reactions after the challenge (Table 4.1) [38].

Data from the severe anaphylaxis literature also indicate that patients who require >1 dose of epinephrine treatment [12, 39–43], fluid resuscitation [12, 42], or inhaled β-agonist for respiratory distress (Fig. 4.1) were more likely to develop biphasic reactions [12]. Although there are no data that directly linked age, male sex, or specific allergen triggers to BA, these factors have been found to increase the risk of severe anaphylaxis [30, 44]. For example, data from the European Anaphylaxis Registry found that each year increment of age was associated with 1.6% (CI, 1.4%–1.9%) increase in the odds of experiencing a severe anaphylactic event [30]. Similarly, male sex, drug, and venom culprit allergens were all associated with severe anaphylaxis [30]. Therefore, clinicians should take these factors into account when making treatment decisions or providing anticipatory guidance for patients.

Impact of epinephrine treatment Timely epinephrine administration plays a significant role in the prevention of severe and fatal anaphylaxis [45–48]. Several recent studies found that patients who received intramuscular epinephrine before arrival to ED had much favorable outcome [49–51]. For example, prospective data from the Cross-Canada Anaphylaxis Registry found that epinephrine administration before arrival to ED was the only factor associated with a reduced risk of multiple epinephrine administration in ED (OR, 0.2; 95% CI, 0.0–0.6) [49]. Similarly, Fleming et al. found that children with food-induced anaphylaxis who received epinephrine before arrival to the ED were less likely to be hospitalized (17% vs 43%, $P < 0.001$) or to require additional therapies compared with those who received epinephrine in the ED [50]. Epinephrine also appears to play a critical role in the prevention of biphasic anaphylaxis [52]. Two recent pediatric and adult studies have found that patients who received intramuscular epinephrine therapy within 60 min of onset of anaphylaxis were at low risk for developing BA [12, 53]. On the other hand, several observational studies have found that epinephrine treatment for initial anaphylaxis was either underused or delayed in patients who developed biphasic reactions [12, 42, 54–58].

Corticosteroids and the risk of biphasic reactions Corticosteroids (CS) are often administered in anaphylaxis based on the theory that the anti-inflammatory effects may reduce the risk of a biphasic reaction. However, the evidence to support this practice is lacking. The roles of CS in anaphylaxis, including the prevention of BA, are extensively reviewed in our recent systemic review [29]. To date, out of 25 studies that examined the association of corticosteroids with BA, no study found any benefit in preventing secondary reactions regardless of the administered dose or formulation of CS (Table 10.1). This finding is consistent with a previous meta-analysis of observational studies that examined the predictors of BA and noted no significant association between the use of CS and the risk of a biphasic reaction (pooled OR, 1.52; 95% CI, 0.96–2.43). Furthermore, among over 5000 children who were diagnosed with anaphylaxis at 35 American children's hospitals between 2009 and 2013, corticosteroid administration was not associated with a reduction in ED revisit for allergic reaction within 72 h from the initial visit (aOR, 1.01; 95% CI, 0.50–2.05) [59].

What is more concerning, though, is the potential harm of CS. The randomized trial by De Silva et al. found that the concomitant administration of hydrocortisone with epinephrine to prevent anaphylaxis from snake antivenom resulted in increasing the risk of a severe reaction [60]. Furthermore, a recent Canadian study assessed the outcome of prehospital treatment with CS among a cohort of close to 3500 children who presented to ED with anaphylactic reactions [61]. CS was found to be associated with increased risk of admission to the ICU or the hospital ward (aOR, 2.88; 95% CI, 1.13, 7.36) and severe reactions (aOR, 11.50; 95% CI, 4.51, 29.33) while adjusting for anaphylaxis severity, treatment with epinephrine and antihistamines, asthma, sex, and age [61].

Gaps in Anaphylaxis Management and Post-anaphylaxis Care

In 2014 the World Allergy Organization research agenda recognized significant knowledge gaps in understanding BA and called for large prospective cohort studies to bridge these gaps for clinical practice [62, 63]. Reflecting the knowledge gaps, guidelines from national and international allergy organizations vary widely in recommendations for post-anaphylaxis care [64–66]. Scope of practice variation for post-anaphylaxis care across developed countries starkly illustrates the impact of this lack of evidence. The 2016 British National Institute for Health and Care Excellence guidelines recommend that all children with anaphylaxis be hospitalized for at least 24 h [65]. Recent data from >30 US children's hospitals showed that up to 50% of children evaluated in EDs for anaphylaxis between 2007 and 2013 were admitted to the hospital [67, 68]. In contrast, Canada's admission rate is around 5% [15, 69].

The practice of admitting all patients appears to add little to patient safety. Of children hospitalized for anaphylaxis, 84% need no further interventions, and symptoms resolve in the ED for 92% [70]. Furthermore, hospitalizations account for the most substantial part of US annual direct medical costs ($1.9 billion) of children with food allergy [71]. Several US hospitals have now implemented local quality measures to reduce anaphylaxis-related admissions [72, 73]. With increasing ED crowding and increasing ED visits for anaphylaxis, the practice of prolonged monitoring of all patients appears neither sustainable nor cost-effective [74]. Updated 2015 anaphylaxis practice parameters moved from universal monitoring for 4–8 h to individualizing the monitoring period [66]. However, BA is a fundamental patient safety concern, and without a validated risk stratification model, this recommendation gives no guidance to clinicians.

Implications for Clinical Practice

- Biphasic anaphylactic reactions are more likely to occur in moderate to severe anaphylaxis or when anaphylaxis is not treated with timely epinephrine. Therefore, the single most effective therapy that could prevent severe and BA is the prompt administration of intramuscular epinephrine.
- Due to the potential detrimental adverse effects of corticosteroids and lack of compelling evidence demonstrating an effective role in reducing anaphylaxis severity or preventing biphasic anaphylaxis, the routine therapy with corticosteroids is not recommended.
- Although data from randomized clinical trials are lacking, patients with refractory anaphylactic shock, severe airway obstruction, or concomitant asthma exacerbation may potentially benefit from corticosteroid therapy.
- After an anaphylactic reaction, the ED monitoring period should be based on the individual patient risk factors for severe anaphylaxis and the presence of aggravating factors (Fig. 4.1). Patient with mild anaphylaxis that remains asymptomatic after one dose of timely epinephrine can be discharged after 4 h [75].
- Prolonged (6–8 h) or overnight monitoring should be considered for any of the following indications:
  1. Anaphylaxis that resolves after two doses of epinephrine therapy
  2. Patients who present to ED late in the evening
  3. Patients who live alone, remote from emergency care, or have no immediate access to an epinephrine auto-injector
  4. Patients with a history of severe or current uncontrolled asthma
- Admission to the hospital for at least 24-h monitoring should be considered for any of the following:
  1. Presentation with severe anaphylaxis (e.g., anaphylactic shock, severe respiratory distress)
  2. Refractory anaphylaxis
  3. Anaphylaxis that requires >2 doses of epinephrine
  4. Drug-induced anaphylaxis

References

1. Simons FER, Ardusso LRF, Bilò MB, El-Gamal YM, Ledford DK, Ring J, et al. World allergy organization guidelines for the assessment and management of anaphylaxis. World Allergy Organ J. 2011;4(2):13–37.
2. Castells M. Diagnosis and management of anaphylaxis in precision medicine. J Allergy Clin Immunol [Internet]. 2017;140(2):321–33. Available from: https://doi.org/10.1016/j.jaci.2017.06.012.
3. Lieberman P. Biphasic anaphylactic reactions. Ann Allergy Asthma Immunol [Internet]. 2005;95(3):217–26; quiz 226, 258. Available from: http://www.ncbi.nlm.nih.gov/pubmed/16200811.
4. Tole JW, Lieberman P. Biphasic anaphylaxis: review of incidence, clinical predictors, and observation recommendations. Immunol Allergy Clin North Am [Internet]. 2007;27(2):309–26, viii. Available from: http://www.ncbi.nlm.nih.gov/pubmed/17493505.
5. Alqurashi W, Ellis AK. Do corticosteroids prevent biphasic anaphylaxis? J Allergy Clin Immunol Pract [Internet]. 2017 [cited 2017 Sep 12];5(5):1194–205. Available from: http://www.ncbi.nlm.nih.gov/pubmed/28888249.
6. Stark BJ, Sullivan TJ. Biphasic and protracted anaphylaxis. J Allergy Clin Immunol [Internet]. 1986;78(1 Pt 1):76–83. Available from: http://www.ncbi.nlm.nih.gov/pubmed/3722636.
7. Lee S, Bellolio MF, Hess EP, Campbell RL. Predictors of biphasic reactions in the emergency department for patients with anaphylaxis. J Allergy Clin Immunol Pract [Internet]. 2014;2(3):281–7. Available from: https://doi.org/10.1016/j.jaip.2014.01.012.
8. Ko BS, Kim WY, Ryoo SM, Ahn S, Sohn CH, Seo DW, et al. Biphasic reactions in patients with anaphylaxis treated with corticosteroids. Ann Allergy Asthma Immunol [Internet]. 2015;115(4):312–6. Available from: http://www.ncbi.nlm.nih.gov/pubmed/26276313.
9. Sugiura A, Nakayama T, Takahara M, Sugimoto K, Hattori N, Abe R, et al. Combined use of ECMO and hemodialysis in the case of contrast-induced biphasic anaphylactic shock. Am J Emerg Med [Internet]. 2016 Sep [cited 2017 Feb 19];34(9):1919.e1–1919.e2. Available from: http://linkinghub.elsevier.com/retrieve/pii/S0735675716001194.
10. Niggemann B, Yürek S, Beyer K. Severe anaphylaxis requiring intensive care during oral food challenge-It is not always peanuts. Pediatr Allergy Immunol [Internet]. 2016;7:1–2. Available from: http://doi.wiley.com/10.1111/pai.12676.
11. Douglas DM, Sukenick E, Andrade WP, Brown JS. Biphasic systemic anaphylaxis: an inpatient and outpatient study. J Allergy Clin Immunol [Internet]. 1994;93(6):977–85. Available from: http://www.ncbi.nlm.nih.gov/pubmed/8006319.
12. Alqurashi W, Stiell I, Chan K, Neto G, Alsadoon A, Wells G. Epidemiology and clinical predictors of biphasic reactions in children with anaphylaxis. Ann Allergy Asthma Immunol [Internet]. 2015;115(3):217–223 e2. Available from: http://www.ncbi.nlm.nih.gov/pubmed/26112147.
13. Lee S, Bellolio MF, Hess EP, Erwin P, Murad MH, Campbell RL. Time of onset and predictors of biphasic anaphylactic reactions: a systematic review and meta-analysis. J Allergy Clin Immunol Pr [Internet]. 2015;3(3):402–8. Available from: http://www.ncbi.nlm.nih.gov/pubmed/25680923.
14. Ellis A. Biphasic anaphylaxis: a review of the incidence, characteristics and predictors. Open Allergy J [Internet]. 2010 [cited 2016 Feb 10]; Available from: http://benthamopen.com/contents/pdf/TOALLJ/TOALLJ-3-24.pdf.
15. Alqurashi W. Management of children with anaphylaxis in the emergency department: practice pattern and prediction of biphasic reactions [Internet]. Université d'Ottawa/University of Ottawa; 2015 [cited 2016 Feb 10]. Available from: http://www.ruor.uottawa.ca/handle/10393/32101.
16. Sala-Cunill A, Guilarte M, Cardona V. Phenotypes, endotypes and biomarkers in anaphylaxis: current insights. Curr Opin Allergy Clin Immunol. 2018;18(5):370–6.
17. Brown SG, Stone SF, Fatovich DM, et al. Anaphylaxis: clinical patterns, mediator release, and severity. J Allergy Clin Immunol. 2013;132(5):1141–9.e5.

18. Francis A, Fatovich DM, Arendts G, Macdonald SP, Bosio E, Nagree Y, et al. Serum mast cell tryptase measurements: sensitivity and specificity for a diagnosis of anaphylaxis in emergency department patients with shock or hypoxaemia. Emerg Med Australas. 2018;30(3):366–74.

19. Stone SF, Brown SG. Mediators released during human anaphylaxis. Curr Allergy Asthma Rep [Internet]. 2012;12(1):33–41. Available from: http://www.ncbi.nlm.nih.gov/pubmed/22086296.

20. Sala-Cunill A, Cardona V. Biomarkers of anaphylaxis, beyond tryptase. Curr Opin Allergy Clin Immunol [Internet]. 2015;15(4):329–36. Available from: http://www.ncbi.nlm.nih.gov/pubmed/26110683.

21. Popa VT, Lerner SA. Biphasic systemic anaphylactic reaction: three illustrative cases. Ann Allergy. 1984;53(2):151–5.

22. Yang PC, Berin MC, Yu L, Perdue MH. Mucosal pathophysiology and inflammatory changes in the late phase of the intestinal allergic reaction in the rat. Am J Pathol. 2001;158(2):681–90.

23. Vadas P, Gold M, Perelman B, Liss GM, Lack G, Blyth T, et al. Platelet-activating factor, PAF acetylhydrolase, and severe anaphylaxis. N Engl J Med [Internet]. 2008 [cited 2017 Feb 21];358(1):28–35. Available from: http://www.nejm.org/doi/abs/10.1056/NEJMoa070030.

24. Vadas P. The platelet-activating factor pathway in food allergy and anaphylaxis. Ann Allergy Asthma Immunol [Internet]. 2016;117(5):455–7. Available from: http://linkinghub.elsevier.com/retrieve/pii/S108112061630223X; http://www.ncbi.nlm.nih.gov/pubmed/27788869.

25. Zheng F, Barthel G, Collange O, Montémont C, Thornton SN, Longrois D, et al. Methylene blue and epinephrine: a synergetic association for anaphylactic shock treatment. Crit Care Med [Internet]. 2013 [cited 2017 Feb 21];41(1):195–204. Available from: http://content.wkhealth.com/linkback/openurl?sid=WKPTLP:landingpage&an=00003246-201301000-00022.

26. Vadas P, Perelman B, Liss G. Platelet-activating factor, histamine, and tryptase levels in human anaphylaxis. J Allergy Clin Immunol [Internet]. 2013 [cited 2017 Feb 21];131(1):144–9. Available from: http://www.ncbi.nlm.nih.gov/pubmed/23040367.

27. Vadas P, Perelman B. Effect of epinephrine on platelet-activating factor-stimulated human vascular smooth muscle cells. J Allergy Clin Immunol [Internet]. 2012 [cited 2017 Feb 21];129(5):1329–33. Available from: http://www.ncbi.nlm.nih.gov/pubmed/22460068.

28. Choi I-W, Kim Y-S, Kim D-K, Choi J-H, Seo K-H, Im S-Y, et al. Platelet-activating factor-mediated NF-kappaB dependency of a late anaphylactic reaction. J Exp Med. 2003;198(1):145–51.

29. Alqurashi W, Ellis AK. Do corticosteroids prevent biphasic anaphylaxis? J Allergy Clin Immunol Pract [Internet]. 2017;5(September 2017):1–12. Available from: https://doi.org/10.1016/j.jaip.2017.05.022.

30. Worm M, Francuzik W, Renaudin J-M, Bilo MB, Cardona V, Hofmeier KS, et al. Factors increasing the risk for a severe reaction in anaphylaxis: an analysis of data from the European anaphylaxis registry. Allergy. 2018;

31. Smith PK, Hourihane JO, Lieberman P. Risk multipliers for severe food anaphylaxis. World Allergy Organ J [Internet]. 2015;8(1):30. Available from: http://www.waojournal.org/content/8/1/30.

32. Hompes S, Kohli A, Nemat K, Scherer K, Lange L, Rueff F, et al. Provoking allergens and treatment of anaphylaxis in children and adolescents--data from the anaphylaxis registry of German-speaking countries. Pediatr Allergy Immunol [Internet]. 2011;22(6):568–74. Available from: http://www.ncbi.nlm.nih.gov/pubmed/21435004.

33. Simons FER, Ardusso LRF, Bilò MB, El-Gamal YM, Ledford DK, Ring J, et al. World allergy organization guidelines for the assessment and management of anaphylaxis. World Allergy Organ J [Internet]. 2011;4(2):13–37. Available from: http://www.ncbi.nlm.nih.gov/pubmed/23268454.

34. Niggemann B, Beyer K. Factors augmenting allergic reactions. Allergy [Internet]. 2014;69(12):1582–7. Available from: http://www.ncbi.nlm.nih.gov/pubmed/25306896.

35. Brown SG. The pathophysiology of shock in anaphylaxis. Immunol Allergy Clin North Am. 2007;27(2):165–75, v.

36. Brown SG, Blackman KE, Stenlake V, Heddle RJ. Insect sting anaphylaxis; prospective evaluation of treatment with intravenous adrenaline and volume resuscitation. Emerg Med J. 2004;21(2):149–54.

37. Pumphrey RS. Lessons for management of anaphylaxis from a study of fatal reactions. Clin Exp Allergy. 2000;30(8):1144–50.
38. Saleh-Langenberg J, Flokstra-De Blok BMJ, Alagla N, Kollen BJ, Dubois AEJ. Late reactions in food-allergic children and adolescents after double-blind, placebo-controlled food challenges. Allergy Eur J Allergy Clin Immunol. 2016;71(7):1069–73.
39. Kim TH, Yoon SH, Lee SY, Choi YH, Park CM, Kang HR, et al. Biphasic and protracted anaphylaxis to iodinated contrast media. Eur Radiol. 2018;28(3):1242–52.
40. Brazil E, MacNamara AF. "Not so immediate" hypersensitivity--the danger of biphasic anaphylactic reactions. J Accid Emerg Med [Internet]. 1998;15(4):252–3. Available from: http://www.ncbi.nlm.nih.gov/pubmed/9681309.
41. Scranton SE, Gonzalez EG, Waibel KH. Incidence and characteristics of biphasic reactions after allergen immunotherapy. J Allergy Clin Immunol [Internet]. 2009;123(2):493–8. Available from: http://www.ncbi.nlm.nih.gov/pubmed/19064282.
42. Mehr S, Liew WK, Tey D, Tang ML. Clinical predictors for biphasic reactions in children presenting with anaphylaxis. Clin Exp Allergy [Internet]. 2009;39(9):1390–6. Available from: http://www.ncbi.nlm.nih.gov/pubmed/19486033.
43. Inoue N, Yamamoto A. Clinical evaluation of pediatric anaphylaxis and the necessity for multiple doses of epinephrine. Asia Pac Allergy. 2013;3(2):106–14.
44. Turner PJ, Jerschow E, Umasunthar T, Lin R, Campbell DE, Boyle RJ. Fatal anaphylaxis: mortality rate and risk factors. J Allergy Clin Immunol Pract [Internet]. 2017;5(5):1169–78. Available from: http://linkinghub.elsevier.com/retrieve/pii/S2213219817305159.
45. Bock SA, Munoz-Furlong A, Sampson HA. Further fatalities caused by anaphylactic reactions to food, 2001-2006. J Allergy Clin Immunol [Internet]. 2007;119(4):1016–8. Available from: http://www.ncbi.nlm.nih.gov/pubmed/17306354.
46. Pumphrey RS, Gowland MH. Further fatal allergic reactions to food in the United Kingdom, 1999–2006. J Allergy Clin Immunol. 2007;119(4):1018–9.
47. Simons FE, Clark S, Camargo CA Jr. Anaphylaxis in the community: learning from the survivors. J Allergy Clin Immunol. 2009;124(2):301–6.
48. Ko BS, Kim JY, Seo D-W, Kim WY, Lee JH, Sheikh A, et al. Should adrenaline be used in patients with hemodynamically stable anaphylaxis? Incident case control study nested within a retrospective cohort study. Sci Rep [Internet]. 2016 [cited 2017 Feb 20];6:20168. Available from: http://www.nature.com/articles/srep20168.
49. Hochstadter E, Clarke A, De Schryver S, LaVieille S, Alizadehfar R, Joseph L, et al. Increasing visits for anaphylaxis and the benefits of early epinephrine administration: a 4-year study at a pediatric emergency department in Montreal, Canada. J Allergy Clin Immunol [Internet]. 2016 [cited 2016 Jun 24];137(6):1888-1890.e4. Available from: http://www.ncbi.nlm.nih.gov/pubmed/27106202.
50. Fleming JT, Clark S, Camargo CA Jr, Rudders SA. Early treatment of food-induced anaphylaxis with epinephrine is associated with a lower risk of hospitalization. J Allergy Clin Immunol Pr [Internet]. 2015;3(1):57–62. Available from: http://www.ncbi.nlm.nih.gov/pubmed/25577619.
51. Ito K, Ono M, Kando N, Matsui T, Nakagawa T, Sugiura S, et al. Surveillance of the use of adrenaline auto-injectors in Japanese children. Allergol Int [Internet]. 2017;2–7. Available from: https://doi.org/10.1016/j.alit.2017.07.002.
52. Ellis AK. Priority role of epinephrine in anaphylaxis further underscored--the impact on biphasic anaphylaxis. Ann Allergy Asthma Immunol [Internet]. 2015 [cited 2016 Feb 10];115(3):165. Available from: http://www.ncbi.nlm.nih.gov/pubmed/26356586.
53. Lee S, Peterson A, Lohse CM, Hess EP, Campbell RL. Further evaluation of factors that may predict biphasic reactions in emergency department anaphylaxis patients. J Allergy Clin Immunol Pract [Internet]. 2017;5(5):1295–301. Available from: https://doi.org/10.1016/j.jaip.2017.07.020.
54. Lee JM, Greenes DS. Biphasic anaphylactic reactions in pediatrics. Pediatrics. 2000;106(4):762–6.
55. Lertnawapan R, Maek-a-nantawat W. Anaphylaxis and biphasic phase in Thailand: 4-year observation. Allergol Int [Internet]. 2011;60(3):283–9. Available from: http://ovidsp.ovid.com/ovidweb.cgi?T=JS&CSC=Y&NEWS=N&PAGE=fulltext&D=medl&AN=21364308.

56. Manuyakorn W, Benjaponpitak S, Kamchaisatian W, Vilaiyuk S, Sasisakulporn C, Jotikasthira W. Pediatric anaphylaxis: triggers, clinical features, and treatment in a tertiary-care hospital. Asian Pacific J Allergy Immunol. 2015;33(4):281–8.

57. Poachanukoon O, Paopairochanakorn C. Incidence of anaphylaxis in the emergency department: a 1-year study in a university hospital. Asian Pac J Allergy Immunol [Internet]. 2006;24(2–3):111–6. Available from: http://www.ncbi.nlm.nih.gov/pubmed/17136875.

58. Ellis AK, Day JH. Incidence and characteristics of biphasic anaphylaxis: a prospective evaluation of 103 patients. Ann Allergy Asthma Immunol [Internet]. 2007;98(1):64–9. Available from: http://www.ncbi.nlm.nih.gov/pubmed/17225722.

59. Michelson KA, Monuteaux MC, Neuman MI. Glucocorticoids and hospital length of stay for children with anaphylaxis: a retrospective study. J Pediatr [Internet]. 2015;167(3):713–9. Available from: http://www.ncbi.nlm.nih.gov/pubmed/26095285.

60. de Silva HAJHJAJ, Pathmeswaran A, Ranasinha CD, Jayamanne S, Samarakoon SB, Hittharage A, et al. Low-dose adrenaline, promethazine, and hydrocortisone in the prevention of acute adverse reactions to antivenom following snakebite: a randomised, double-blind, placebo-controlled trial. Winkel K, editor. PLoS Med [Internet]. 2011 [cited 2017 Feb 22];8(5):e1000435. Available from: http://dx.plos.org/10.1371/journal.pmed.1000435.

61. Gabrielli S, Clarke A, Morris J, Eisman H, Gravel J, Enarson P, et al. Evaluation of prehospital management in a Canadian emergency department anaphylaxis cohort. J Allergy Clin Immunol Pract. 2019;7(7):2232–8.e3.

62. Simons FER, Ardusso LR, Bilò MB, Cardona V, Ebisawa M, El-Gamal YM, et al. International consensus on (ICON) anaphylaxis. World Allergy Organ J [Internet]. 2014;7(1):9. Available from: http://www.ncbi.nlm.nih.gov/pubmed/24920969.

63. Muraro A, Roberts G, Worm M, Bilo MB, Brockow K, Fernandez Rivas M, et al. Anaphylaxis: guidelines from the European academy of allergy and clinical immunology. Allergy [Internet]. 2014;69(8):1026–45. Available from: http://www.ncbi.nlm.nih.gov/pubmed/24909803.

64. Canadian Society of Allergy and Clinical Immunology. Anaphylaxis in schools & other settings [Internet]. 2016 [cited 2016 Dec 10]. Available from: http://csaci.ca/wp-content/uploads/2017/11/Anaphylaxis-in-Schools-Other-Settings-3rd-Edition-Revised_a.pdf.

65. National Institute for Health and Clinical Excellence. Anaphylaxis: assessment and referral after emergency treatment | Guidance and guidelines | NICE [Internet]. NICE; 2016 [cited 2016 Dec 12]. Available from: https://www.nice.org.uk/guidance/cg134/chapter/4-Research-recommendations#the-frequency-and-effects-of-biphasic-reactions.

66. Lieberman P, Nicklas RA, Randolph C, Oppenheimer J, Bernstein D, Bernstein J, et al. Anaphylaxis-a practice parameter update 2015. Ann Allergy Asthma Immunol [Internet]. 2015;115(5):341–84. Available from: http://www.ncbi.nlm.nih.gov/pubmed/26505932.

67. Parlaman JP, Oron AP, Uspal NG, DeJong KN, Tieder JS. Emergency and hospital care for food-related anaphylaxis in children. Hosp Pediatr. 2016;6(5):269–74.

68. Michelson KA, Monuteaux MC, Neuman MI. Variation and trends in anaphylaxis care in United States Children's hospitals. Acad Emerg Med. 2016;23(5):623–7.

69. Lee AY, Enarson P, Clarke AE, La Vieille S, Eisman H, Chan ES, et al. Anaphylaxis across two Canadian pediatric centers: evaluating management disparities. J Asthma Allergy [Internet]. 2017 [cited 2017 Mar 9];10:1–7. Available from: https://www.dovepress.com/anaphylaxis-across-two-canadian-pediatric-centers-evaluating-managemen-peer-reviewed-article-JAA.

70. Rudders SA, Clark S, Camargo CA. Inpatient interventions are infrequent during pediatric hospitalizations for food-induced anaphylaxis. J Allergy Clin Immunol Pract [Internet]. 2017;5(5):1421–1424. e2. Available from: http://linkinghub.elsevier.com/retrieve/pii/S2213219817303525.

71. Gupta R, Holdford D, Bilaver L, Dyer A, Holl JL, Meltzer D. The economic impact of childhood food allergy in the United States. JAMA Pediatr. 2013;167(11):1026–31.

72. Farbman KS, Michelson KA, Neuman MI, Dribin TE, Schneider LC, Stack AM. Reducing hospitalization rates for children with anaphylaxis. Pediatrics [Internet]. 2017;139(6):e20164114. Available from: http://pediatrics.aappublications.org/lookup/doi/10.1542/peds.2016-4114.

73. Desai SH, Jeong K, Kattan JD, Lieberman R, Wisniewski S, Green TD. Anaphylaxis management before and after implementation of guidelines in the pediatric emergency department. J Allergy Clin Immunol Pract. 3(4):604–606.e2.

74. Grunau BE, Li J, Yi TW, Stenstrom R, Grafstein E, Wiens MO, et al. Incidence of clinically important biphasic reactions in emergency department patients with allergic reactions or anaphylaxis. Ann Emerg Med [Internet]. 2014;63(6):736–744.e2. Available from: https://doi.org/10.1016/j.annemergmed.2013.10.017.

75. TRanslating Emergency Knowledge for Kids (TREKK). Bottom Line Recommendations: Anaphylaxis. [Internet]. 2018. Available from: https://trekk.ca/system/assets/assets/attachments/338/original/2018-12-14_Anaphylaxis_BLR_version_1.2.pdf?1545083199.

76. Sampson HA, Mendelson L, Rosen JP. Fatal and near-fatal anaphylactic reactions to food in children and adolescents. N Engl J Med. 1992;327(6):380–4.

77. Brady WJ Jr, Luber S, Carter CT, Guertler A, Lindbeck G. Multiphasic anaphylaxis: an uncommon event in the emergency department. Acad Emerg Med. 1997;4(3):193–7.

78. Smit DV, Cameron PA, Rainer TH. Anaphylaxis presentations to an emergency department in Hong Kong: incidence and predictors of biphasic reactions. J Emerg Med [Internet]. 2005;28(4):381–8. Available from: http://www.ncbi.nlm.nih.gov/pubmed/15837017.

79. Jirapongsananuruk O, Bunsawansong W, Piyaphanee N, Visitsunthorn N, Thongngarm T, Vichyanond P. Features of patients with anaphylaxis admitted to a university hospital. Ann Allergy Asthma Immunol [Internet]. 2007;98(2):157–62. Available from: http://www.ncbi.nlm.nih.gov/pubmed/17304883.

80. Confino-Cohen R, Goldberg A. Allergen immunotherapy-induced biphasic systemic reactions: incidence, characteristics, and outcome: a prospective study. Ann Allergy Asthma Immunol [Internet]. 2010;104(1):73–8. Available from: http://www.ncbi.nlm.nih.gov/pubmed/20143649.

81. Orhan F, Canitez Y, Bakirtas A, Yilmaz O, Boz AB, Can D, et al. Anaphylaxis in Turkish children: a multi-centre, retrospective, case study. Clin Exp Allergy [Internet]. 2011;41(12):1767–76. Available from: http://www.ncbi.nlm.nih.gov/pubmed/22092675.

82. Lee J, Garrett JP-D, Brown-Whitehorn T, Spergel JM. Biphasic reactions in children undergoing oral food challenges. Allergy Asthma Proc. 2013;34(3):220–6.

83. Nagano C, Ishiguro A, Yotani N, Sakai H, Fujiwara T, Ohya Y. Anaphylaxis and biphasic reaction in a children hospital. Arerugi - Japanese J Allergol [Internet]. 2013;62(2):163–70. Available from: http://ovidsp.ovid.com/ovidweb.cgi?T=JS&CSC=Y&NEWS=N&PAGE=fulltext&D=prem&AN=23531652

84. Vezir E, Erkocoglu M, Kaya A, Toyran M, Ozcan C, Akan A, et al. Characteristics of anaphylaxis in children referred to a tertiary care center. Allergy Asthma Proc. 2013;34(3):239–46.

85. Liew WK, Chiang WC, Goh AE, Lim HH, Chay OM, Chang S, et al. Paediatric anaphylaxis in a Singaporean children cohort: changing food allergy triggers over time, Asia Pac Allergy [Internet]. 2013;3(1):29–34. Available from: http://www.ncbi.nlm.nih.gov/pubmed/23403810.

86. Rohacek M, Edenhofer H, Bircher A, Bingisser R. Biphasic anaphylactic reactions: occurrence and mortality. Allergy [Internet]. 2014;69(6):791–7. Available from: http://www.ncbi.nlm.nih.gov/pubmed/24725226.

87. Oya S, Nakamori T, Kinoshita H. Incidence and characteristics of biphasic and protracted anaphylaxis: evaluation of 114 inpatients. Acute Med Surg. 2014;1(4):228–33.

88. Sricharoen P, Sittichanbuncha Y, Wibulpolprasert A, Srabongkosh E, Sawanyawisuth K. What clinical factors are associated with biphasic anaphylaxis in Thai adult patients? Asian Pacific J Allergy Immunol. 2015;33(1):8–13.

89. Dribin TE, Michelson KA, Monuteaux MC, Stack AM, Farbman KS, Schneider LC, et al. Identification of children with anaphylaxis at low risk of receiving acute inpatient therapies. PLoS One [Internet]. 2019;14(2):1–12. Available from: https://doi.org/10.1371/journal.pone.0211949.

Exercise-Induced Anaphylaxis

5

Babak Aberumand and Anne K. Ellis

Definition

Exercise-induced anaphylaxis (EIA) is defined as a physical allergic reaction with symptoms of anaphylaxis involving four main organ systems: the respiratory tract, the cardiovascular system, the skin, and the gastrointestinal tract after physical activity [1]. With the respiratory tract, symptoms include wheezing, hoarseness of voice, or laryngeal edema, whereas symptoms related to the cardiovascular system include hypotension, chest tightness, weakness, dizziness, and syncope. In terms of the skin, there can be flushing, generalized pruritus with urticaria, and angioedema. Furthermore, common symptoms involving the gastroenterology intact include cramping, nausea, vomiting, and diarrhea [1, 2]. EIA was first described in 1980 when characteristic features of anaphylaxis were noted after exercise in 23 patients over a 10-year period, similar to anaphylaxis elicited by ingestion of an allergen [1]. Since then, the type of physical activity capable of triggering this syndrome has been found to vary and may not always result in anaphylaxis if repeated by the same patient [1, 3]. EIA can occur in all ages and does not have a predilection for sex [4]. It has been reported in varying levels of active individuals from high-performance athletes to those that only occasionally exercise [5]. Although there is heterogeneity in individuals susceptible to EIA, atopy has been found to be a related condition [1, 2]. Extreme temperatures such as warm or cold environments and high humidity have also been found to be associated with EIA [1, 6].

Pathophysiology

The mechanism of EIA is not completely understood. Several hypotheses have been proposed.

B. Aberumand · A. K. Ellis (✉)
Queen's University, Kingston, ON, Canada
e-mail: 0ba11@queensu.ca; Anne.Ellis@kingstonhsc.ca

© Springer Nature Switzerland AG 2020
A. K. Ellis (ed.), *Anaphylaxis*, https://doi.org/10.1007/978-3-030-43205-8_5

Wolanczyk-Medrala et al. found that increased basophil histamine release occurred from physical effort that resulted in a transient serum hyperosmolarity after exposure to a sensitizing food allergen in a patient with FDEIA. They used histamine release assays that detected an increase in histamine release only in FDEIA patients with a buffer osmolarity of 340 mOsm and not levels of 280 mOsm or 450 mOsm [7]. This led to a subsequent study to determine the significance of increased medium osmolarity, which was found to partially mimic circumstances of vigorous physical exercise, on basophil activation. They found that only FDEIA patients had significantly increased in basophil activity in slightly elevated medium osmolarity (340 mOsm), which the authors suggest might be among the factors predisposing to the occurrence of FDEIA. However, the findings in these studies should be taken with caution given the small sample sizes and that such high osmolality levels might not be attained through robust physical activity [8]. A plasma osmolarity of 311 ± 2.4 mOsm has been reported after performing a constant work rate exercise test (60 rpm at 50% of their determined VO2 peak) for 30 minutes [9].

Another proposed mechanism for FDEIA hinges on changes in serum pH whereby a decrease in blood pH triggered mast cell degranulation and pretreatment with sodium bicarbonate prevented symptoms of FDEIA during exercise [10, 11]. In one patient with EIA, several provocation tests done in 2-week intervals were done to produce the symptoms of EIA and the patient was given either 3 g of PO sodium bicarbonate 10 minutes before exercise or placebo (lactose). When given 3 g of PO sodium bicarbonate, the patient had no symptoms of EIA, and their spirometry results were normal. The other patient with EIA, a professional bicyclist, refused provocation and was given 3 g of PO sodium bicarbonate prior to exercise and was found to have no symptoms of EIA while exercising [10]. In a patient with wheat-dependent EIA, pretreatment with sodium bicarbonate inhibited the reoccurrence of anaphylaxis following wheat and exercise provocation. There was also no elevation in plasma histamine level [11].

In patients with wheat-dependent EIA, it has also been proposed that tissue transglutaminase (tTG), an enzyme found beneath the single-layer epithelium of the gastrointestinal tract, plays a role in cross-linking ω-5 gliadin (Tri a 19), a major allergen identified in wheat-dependent EIA [12–14]. This intracellular enzyme is normally dormant in terms of cross-linking during normal physiologic conditions [15]. However, when the body is under stress such as during physical exercise, tTG's cross-linking potential is activated [16–18]. Upregulation of tTG is achieved through an increase in the inflammatory mediator interleukin-6 (IL-6), which is upregulated in exercise through contracting skeletal muscles [19–21]. ω-5 gliadin (Tri a 19) is retained after exposure to gastrointestinal digestive enzymes such as pepsin and trypsin and consequently interacts with tTG after absorption through the gut epithelium. The cross-linking between ω-5 gliadin (Tri a 19) and tTG forms high-molecular-weight complexes that significantly increase IgE binding in patients with wheat-dependent EIA and, as a result, are capable of eliciting an anaphylactic reaction in sensitized individuals [14].

It has been hypothesized that exercise-induced redistribution of blood flow away from the viscera to the skeletal muscle and skin exposes food allergenic peptides to a phenotypically different type of mast cells as compared to the gut. Consequently, the food allergenic peptides are not absorbed in the gut as they would be at rest and concentrate in the skeletal muscle and skin where they have a potential to elicit anaphylaxis [5].

Several studies suggest that exercise in conjunction with aspirin affects the absorption of allergens from the gastrointestinal tract by causing gastrointestinal mucosal damage leading to increased gastrointestinal permeability [22, 23]. This process leads to an increase in the amount of allergen circulating in the blood and increases the potential for an anaphylactic reaction [24, 25]. Matsuo et al. measured the serum gliadin levels of patients with wheat-dependent EIA as well as levels in healthy subjects during provocation tests that included a combination of exercise, wheat ingestion, and aspirin intake and discovered that both groups had an increase in levels of serum gliadin. However, allergic symptoms only occurred in patients with wheat-dependent EIA. The authors hypothesize that the increases of serum gliadin levels by an exercise and aspirin challenge combined with wheat ingestion in both patients with wheat-dependent EIA and healthy subjects suggest that exercise and aspirin assist in the absorption of causative allergens from the gastrointestinal tract into the circulating blood leading to allergic symptoms in FDEIA [26]. However, a study done by *Fordtran and Saltin* on the effects of gastric emptying and intestinal absorption during prolonged severe exercise (1 hour at a relative workload of 71% of maximum) found that even though there was a minor inhibitory effect on gastric emptying, there was no effect on intestinal absorption with exercise. They concluded that gut perfusion and intestinal absorption do not grossly alter mesenteric blood flow during exercise [27].

Antacids and proton pump inhibitors have also been proposed in playing a role by increasing the risk of FDEIA through their mechanism of suppressing acid.

In a case series of patients with FDEIA, it was postulated that exercising decreased gastric acid production via increased sympathetic innervation and decreased mesenteric blood flood. This resulted in a decrease in digestion of allergens allowing the allergen to remain structurally intact as it is absorbed, which may potentially cross the threshold of IgE-mediated mast cell degranulation [28]. This theory was further supported by a murine study that found when antacids such as H2-receptor blockers and proton pump inhibitors (PPIs) were taken with digestion-labile allergens, the allergens induced specific IgE antibodies that elicited a positive mucosal and skin reaction [29]. A follow-up observational cohort study found that 25% of dyspeptic patients taking H2 blockers or PPIs for a period of at least 3 months had de novo IgE formation with associated IgE-mediated allergic symptoms. Sensitization was still present on skin testing 5 months after the discontinuation of the antacids [30]. This suggests that acid suppression via exercise or antacids plays a role in increasing the risk of FDEIA.

In general, EIA may have a multifactorial pathogenesis. However, it does appear to be a mast cell-mediated disorder with temporary elevations in plasma histamine and serum tryptase [31, 32]. The exact triggers for mast cell activation and the relationship to exercise that changes the behavior of mast cells have yet to be fully uncovered and validated.

Clinical Presentation

EIA tends to occur after a short duration of exercise not necessarily requiring full maximal effort. It is a diagnosis made on clinical assessment [5]. Initially there is fatigue, flushing, pruritus, erythema, and urticaria. However with continued exercise, these symptoms shift to angioedema, gastrointestinal upset, laryngeal edema, and/or cardiovascular collapse [1, 4]. Other associated symptoms include wheezing that is not as common as in exercise-induced bronchospasm, nausea, vomiting, diarrhea, abdominal pain, and headache [1].

At least one other co-trigger needs to be present to elicit EIA. These include nonsteroidal anti-inflammatory drugs (NSAIDs), alcoholic beverages, menstruation, or pollen exposure in the pollen-sensitized patient [3, 4, 6, 24, 33]. Food is another common co-trigger, and when involved, it is referred as food-dependent EIA (FDEIA). Common culprit foods associated with food-induced EIA include celery, wheat, tree nuts, and shellfish [2, 4, 33–36]. However, almost any food can be associated with FDEIA [4]. FDEIA patients typically do not react after eating the food without exercising. They also do not usually react if they exercise first and then eat the food. More often than not, if they eat the food and then exercise, they will have an anaphylactic reaction [3, 36]. However, it has been reported that a patient developed FDEIA after first exercising and then eating celery [2]. When the food allergen is ingested exclusively or the exercise occurs exclusively, they are tolerated by patients with FDEIA [5]. Typically the ingestion of food or alcohol must occur 4–6 hours prior to exercising, whereas NSAIDs can be taken up to 24 hours, in order for a reaction to occur [3]. FDEIA patients tend to have a mixed presentation of a food antigen-induced anaphylaxis and exercise-related anaphylactic syndrome [2].

Diagnosis

The differential diagnosis of EIA includes arrhythmias, vocal dysfunction, exercise-induced bronchoconstriction, and cholinergic urticaria [3]. Exercise-induced bronchoconstriction, formally known as exercise-induced asthma, differs from EIA in that the hallmark symptom is wheezing. The wheezing occurs during or more commonly after exercise in the absence of other allergic symptoms such as urticaria and angioedema [2, 5]. Having asthma is not a prerequisite for exercise-induced bronchoconstriction, though up to 90% of patients that develop exercise-induced bronchoconstriction will have asthma [37].

Cholinergic urticaria, on the other hand, is thought to be a heat-induced syndrome whereby symptoms typically occur with hot showers and hot weather conditions. The heat from rigorous exercise has been reported to induce cholinergic urticaria. The urticarial lesions of cholinergic urticaria differ from those of EIA as they are much smaller (1–2 mm), appear initially on the neck and thorax, and are reproducible by an intradermal injection of methacholine [2].

A controlled exercise challenge such as a treadmill test can be used to elicit the symptoms of EIA [3]. It will also cause a rise in levels of serum histamine and serum tryptase compared to those without EIA [31, 32]. However this challenge test is limited in that it does not consistently produce symptoms [31, 38]. Importantly, exercise must occur in order for the diagnosis to be EIA, and the identification of potential co-triggers through the clinical history plays a crucial role in making the diagnosis [3]. A diagnosis of FDEIA must be excluded before a diagnosis of EIA can be made [5].

Management

The management of EIA does not differ from other forms of anaphylaxis, and prompt administration of epinephrine is warranted. Resolution of cutaneous manifestations of EIA can be achieved through the administration of antihistamines. Patients with persistent hypotension or evident laryngeal edema should be transferred to a monitored high-acuity facility where vasoactive medications, oxygen, and an emergency airway can be obtained [1]. Once the patient stops exercising or treatment is administered, symptom resolution is achieved quite rapidly within a few hours. Patients with EIA must carry two epinephrine auto-injectors at all times and should be encouraged to exercise in a supervised setting where someone can help administer epinephrine should an anaphylactic reaction occur. Advising patients on avoiding identified cofactors that are not limited to eating specific foods, NSAIDs, and certain weather conditions will allow them to exercise without developing a reaction [1, 3].

Prevention

Medications used prophylactically, such as pretreatment with antihistamines, have not shown to universally prevent symptoms of EIA [3, 4]. However, protective effects with cetirizine and montelukast have been reported in FDEIA [39]. Pretreatment with mast cell stabilizers such as ketotifen has also shown promise [40, 41]. It is important to note that strong evidence is currently lacking for these medications [3]. Pretreatment with sodium bicarbonate 3 g has also been suggested to prevent anaphylaxis in patients with EIA or FDEIA [10, 11]. Counseling patients on stopping exercise immediately if they start developing symptoms as continued exercise can worsen symptoms is the mainstay of prevention. Patients should be encouraged to continue to exercise and live an active lifestyle but with modifications to minimize the risk of eliciting another anaphylactic attack [1].

References

1. Sheffer AL, Austen KF. Exercise-induced anaphylaxis. J Allergy Clin Immunol. 1980;66(2):106–11.
2. Kidd JM 3rd, Cohen SH, Sosman AJ, Fink JN. Food-dependent exercise-induced anaphylaxis. J Allergy Clin Immunol. 1983;71(4):407–11.
3. Lieberman P, Nicklas RA, Randolph C, Oppenheimer J, Bernstein D, Bernstein J, et al. Anaphylaxis--a practice parameter update 2015. Ann Allergy Asthma Immunol. 2015;115(5):341–84.

4. Shadick NA, Liang MH, Partridge AJ, Bingham IC, Wright E, Fossel AH, et al. The natural history of exercise-induced anaphylaxis: survey results from a 10-year follow-up study. J Allergy Clin Immunol. 1999;104(1):123–7.

5. Robson-Ansley P, Toit GD. Pathophysiology, diagnosis and management of exercise-induced anaphylaxis. Curr Opin Allergy Clin Immunol. 2010;10(4):312–7.

6. Wade JP, Liang MH, Sheffer AL. Exercise-induced anaphylaxis: epidemiologic observations. Prog Clin Biol Res. 1989;297:175–82.

7. Barg W, Wolanczyk-Medrala A, Obojski A, Wytrychowski K, Panaszek B, Medrala W. Food-dependent exercise-induced anaphylaxis: possible impact of increased basophil histamine releasability in hyperosmolar conditions. J Investig Allergol Clin Immunol. 2008;18(4):312–5.

8. Wolanczyk-Medrala A, Barg W, Gogolewski G, Panaszek B, Liebhart J, Litwa M, et al. Influence of hyperosmotic conditions on basophil CD203c upregulation in patients with food-dependent exercise-induced anaphylaxis. Ann Agric Environ Med. 2009;16(2):301–4.

9. Khamnei S, Alipour MR, Ahmadiasl N. The combined effects of exercise and post dehydration water drinking on plasma arginine vasopressin, plasma osmolality and body temperature in healthy males. Int J Endocrinol Metab. 2005;2:80–6.

10. Azofra Garcia J, Sastre Dominguez J, Olaguibel Rivera JM, Hernandez de Rojas D, Estupinan Saltos M, Sastre Castillo A. Exercise-induced anaphylaxis: inhibition with sodium bicarbonate. Allergy. 1986;41(6):471.

11. Katsunuma T, Iikura Y, Akasawa A, Iwasaki A, Hashimoto K, Akimoto K. Wheat-dependent exercise-induced anaphylaxis: inhibition by sodium bicarbonate. Ann Allergy. 1992;68(2):184–8.

12. Molberg O, McAdam SN, Korner R, Quarsten H, Kristiansen C, Madsen L, et al. Tissue transglutaminase selectively modifies gliadin peptides that are recognized by gut-derived T cells in celiac disease. Nat Med. 1998;4(6):713–7.

13. Palosuo K, Alenius H, Varjonen E, Koivuluhta M, Mikkola J, Keskinen H, et al. A novel wheat gliadin as a cause of exercise-induced anaphylaxis. J Allergy Clin Immunol. 1999;103(5 Pt 1):912–7.

14. Palosuo K, Varjonen E, Nurkkala J, Kalkkinen N, Harvima R, Reunala T, et al. Transglutaminase-mediated cross-linking of a peptic fraction of omega-5 gliadin enhances IgE reactivity in wheat-dependent, exercise-induced anaphylaxis. J Allergy Clin Immunol. 2003;111(6):1386–92.

15. Smethurst PA, Griffin M. Measurement of tissue transglutaminase activity in a permeabilized cell system: its regulation by Ca2+ and nucleotides. Biochem J. 1996;313(Pt 3):803–8.

16. Korner G, Deutsch VR, Vlodavsky I, Eldor A. Effects of ionizing irradiation on endothelial cell transglutaminase. FEBS Lett. 1993;330(1):41–5.

17. Kim SY, Jeitner TM, Steinert PM. Transglutaminases in disease. Neurochem Int. 2002;40(1):85–103.

18. Hoffman-Goetz L, Pedersen BK. Exercise and the immune system: a model of the stress response? Immunol Today. 1994;15(8):382–7.

19. Suto N, Ikura K, Sasaki R. Expression induced by interleukin-6 of tissue-type transglutaminase in human hepatoblastoma HepG2 cells. J Biol Chem. 1993;268(10):7469–73.

20. Ostrowski K, Rohde T, Zacho M, Asp S, Pedersen BK. Evidence that interleukin-6 is produced in human skeletal muscle during prolonged running. J Physiol. 1998;508(Pt 3):949–53.

21. Pedersen BK, Steensberg A, Schjerling P. Exercise and interleukin-6. Curr Opin Hematol. 2001;8(3):137–41.

22. Lambert GP, Broussard LJ, Mason BL, Mauermann WJ, Gisolfi CV. Gastrointestinal permeability during exercise: effects of aspirin and energy-containing beverages. J Appl Physiol (1985). 2001;90(6):2075–80.

23. Ryan AJ, Chang RT, Gisolfi CV. Gastrointestinal permeability following aspirin intake and prolonged running. Med Sci Sports Exerc. 1996;28(6):698–705.

24. Harada S, Horikawa T, Ashida M, Kamo T, Nishioka E, Ichihashi M. Aspirin enhances the induction of type I allergic symptoms when combined with food and exercise in patients with food-dependent exercise-induced anaphylaxis. Br J Dermatol. 2001;145(2):336–9.

25. Aihara M, Miyazawa M, Osuna H, Tsubaki K, Ikebe T, Aihara Y, et al. Food-dependent exercise-induced anaphylaxis: influence of concurrent aspirin administration on skin testing and provocation. Br J Dermatol. 2002;146(3):466–72.
26. Matsuo H, Morimoto K, Akaki T, Kaneko S, Kusatake K, Kuroda T, et al. Exercise and aspirin increase levels of circulating gliadin peptides in patients with wheat-dependent exercise-induced anaphylaxis. Clin Exp Allergy. 2005;35(4):461–6.
27. Fordtran JS, Saltin B. Gastric emptying and intestinal absorption during prolonged severe exercise. J Appl Physiol. 1967;23(3):331–5.
28. Chen JY, Quirt J, Lee KJ. Proposed new mechanism for food and exercise induced anaphylaxis based on case studies. Allergy Asthma Clin Immunol. 2013;9(1):11.
29. Untersmayr E, Scholl I, Swoboda I, Beil WJ, Forster-Waldl E, Walter F, et al. Antacid medication inhibits digestion of dietary proteins and causes food allergy: a fish allergy model in BALB/c mice. J Allergy Clin Immunol. 2003;112(3):616–23.
30. Untersmayr E, Bakos N, Scholl I, Kundi M, Roth-Walter F, Szalai K, et al. Anti-ulcer drugs promote IgE formation toward dietary antigens in adult patients. FASEB J. 2005;19(6):656–8.
31. Sheffer AL, Soter NA, McFadden ER Jr, Austen KF. Exercise-induced anaphylaxis: a distinct form of physical allergy. J Allergy Clin Immunol. 1983;71(3):311–6.
32. Schwartz HJ. Elevated serum tryptase in exercise-induced anaphylaxis. J Allergy Clin Immunol. 1995;95(4):917–9.
33. Dohi M, Suko M, Sugiyama H, Yamashita N, Tadokoro K, Juji F, et al. Food-dependent, exercise-induced anaphylaxis: a study on 11 Japanese cases. J Allergy Clin Immunol. 1991;87(1 Pt 1):34–40.
34. Guinnepain MT, Eloit C, Raffard M, Brunet-Moret MJ, Rassemont R, Laurent J. Exercise-induced anaphylaxis: useful screening of food sensitization. Ann Allergy Asthma Immunol. 1996;77(6):491–6.
35. Armentia A, Martin-Santos JM, Blanco M, Carretero L, Puyo M, Barber D. Exercise-induced anaphylactic reaction to grain flours. Ann Allergy. 1990;65(2):149–51.
36. Maulitz RM, Pratt DS, Schocket AL. Exercise-induced anaphylactic reaction to shellfish. J Allergy Clin Immunol. 1979;63(6):433–4.
37. McFadden ER Jr, Gilbert IA. Exercise-induced asthma. N Engl J Med. 1994;330(19):1362–7.
38. Romano A, Di Fonso M, Giuffreda F, Papa G, Artesani MC, Viola M, et al. Food-dependent exercise-induced anaphylaxis: clinical and laboratory findings in 54 subjects. Int Arch Allergy Immunol. 2001;125(3):264–72.
39. Peroni DG, Piacentini GL, Piazza M, Cametti E, Boner AL. Combined cetirizine-montelukast preventive treatment for food-dependent exercise-induced anaphylaxis. Ann Allergy Asthma Immunol. 2010;104(3):272–3.
40. Juji F, Suko M. Effectiveness of disodium cromoglycate in food-dependent, exercise-induced anaphylaxis: a case report. Ann Allergy. 1994;72(5):452–4.
41. Choi JH, Lee HB, Ahn IS, Park CW, Lee CH. Wheat-dependent, exercise-induced anaphylaxis: a successful case of prevention with ketotifen. Ann Dermatol. 2009;21(2):203–5.

In-Office Preparedness for Anaphylaxis

Erin Banta and Marcella Aquino

Abbreviations

ACE-Is	Angiotensin-converting enzyme inhibitors
EAI	Epinephrine auto-injector
EMS	Emergency medical services
Ig	Immunoglobulin
IT	Immunotherapy
NL	Normal
NSAIDs	Nonsteroidal anti-inflammatory drugs
ODCs	Oral drug challenges
OFCs	Oral food challenges
SCIT	Subcutaneous immunotherapy
WAO	World Allergy Organization

Introduction

Anaphylaxis is an unpredictable and life-threatening event that can result from commonly performed testing and procedures in the outpatient allergy/immunology setting. Rapid identification of anaphylaxis and its prompt treatment are critical to

E. Banta
NYU Winthrop Hospital, Division of Rheumatology, Allergy & Immunology,
Mineola, NY, USA
e-mail: erin.banta@nyulangone.org

M. Aquino (✉)
Rhode Island Hospital/Hasbro Children's Hospital,
Warren Alpert Medical School of Brown University, Providence, RI, USA
e-mail: maquino@lifespan.org; marcella_aquino@brown.edu

© Springer Nature Switzerland AG 2020
A. K. Ellis (ed.), *Anaphylaxis*, https://doi.org/10.1007/978-3-030-43205-8_6

positive outcomes. Therefore, office preparedness is essential for the appropriate management of anaphylaxis in this setting. Anaphylaxis is a risk associated with subcutaneous immunotherapy (SCIT), skin testing, oral food and drug challenges (OFCs, ODCs), as well as the administration of vaccines, biologics, and immunoglobulin (Ig). Safeguarding against anaphylaxis and its feared adverse outcomes requires preparation for a predictable, timely, and purposeful response. Since a reaction can happen anywhere between the physician's office and the patient's home, both the patient and staff must be aware of the signs and symptoms of anaphylaxis as well as their role in response to these signs. Developing an office action plan for anaphylaxis is recommended as a way to ensure appropriate management [1].

An office action plan to respond to anaphylaxis should include the following parts: education for staff and patients, an anaphylaxis emergency kit or cart including a protocol for treatment, and a mechanism to reinforce, troubleshoot, and update the office plan [1, 2]. Additional procedure-specific safeguards can be considered with regard to patient selection to minimize risks where possible.

Ongoing medical and clerical staff education should be structured, reoccurring, and scheduled, with some sources suggesting this occur every 3 months [1, 2]. The education program developed in an office should be sufficient to give the office manager, front desk staff, medical assistants, nurses, and mid-level providers a working knowledge of the definition of anaphylaxis. These educational endeavors should also identify patients who are at risk for anaphylaxis (e.g., those with uncontrolled medical problems, those on angiotensin-converting enzyme inhibitors [ACE-Is] or β-blocker antihypertensive drugs) [1, 2]. All members of the staff should be aware of which commonly performed procedures in the office might trigger anaphylaxis. Additionally, signs, symptoms, and the spectrum of presentation of anaphylaxis should be part of the education program. Staff must be able to identify anaphylaxis and initiate the office protocol for management so that treatment may begin as quickly as possible. Delay in treatment of anaphylaxis is a major contributing factor to fatalities [3, 4].

Another important facet of the reoccurring education program should include the definition of staff roles when anaphylaxis occurs. The key roles in the treatment of anaphylaxis include reporter (person who identifies problem), leader (clinician directing treatment), medical support (administrator of medications/O_2, obtaining vital sign checks), scribe (documents time/medication administration/patient status), and communications support (often front desk staff responsible for contacting emergency medical services [EMS]). Education for medical support must include a review of the location of supplies used in the treatment of anaphylaxis (emergency anaphylaxis kit). Reoccurring education should also include the review of these supplies to ensure that they are not expired. Key phone numbers should be easily accessible in the event that emergency services are required. Office layout issues (elevator access, clinic obstacles, etc.) should be considered and discussed in a preventative manner rather than confronted during an emergency. Roles may be practiced, and logistical issues anticipated, through the use of mock anaphylaxis office drills discussed later.

Emergency Kit/Cart

All offices that perform procedures associated with a risk of anaphylaxis should have the supplies necessary to treat it and a written emergency protocol or algorithm to direct and document treatment (Fig. 6.1) [1, 2]. This anaphylaxis emergency kit or cart should be easily accessible and, based on expert opinion, is recommended to contain at least first-line treatment supplies, though second-line and third-line supplies should also be considered depending on staff knowledge of their use [1]. The kit or cart should include an inventory sheet with expiration dates for medications, and this can be reviewed every 3 months as part of the office education program. First-line items that should be present in every kit/cart include a stethoscope, sphygmomanometer, injectable epinephrine 1:1000, oxygen, intravenous 0.9% normal (NL) saline, a one-way valve face mask, oropharyngeal and nasopharyngeal airways, disposable face masks, oxygen saturation monitor, albuterol inhalation solution, glucagon, and supplies for administration of all items (large bore needles/tubing supplies/syringes/gloves/tape/antiseptic swabs) [1]. Adjunct supplies vary but typically include the following medications: antihistamines, H2 blockers, and systemic corticosteroids [2, 5], defibrillator, and laryngeal mask airways. The written office protocol or algorithm should direct a detailed, easy-to-follow, stepwise approach to treatment and allow the scribe to easily document each intervention following evidence-based guidelines [1]. It should be posted in all patient care areas and stored with the anaphylaxis emergency kit/cart. The anaphylaxis cart or kit should be mobile so that it can be easily moved to the location of the patient [1].

Documentation of Reactions

The documentation of a reaction occurring in the allergy office is essential. Requirements for documentation include the type of reaction (symptoms, vitals, physical exam findings), trigger allergen (IT, drug or food challenge, biologic, Ig replacement), dosages of medications administered (epinephrine, antihistamines, corticosteroids), and other interventions (intravenous fluid, oxygen). The scribe is responsible for accurate measurements of time: when the reaction was noted, the time that the interventions were administered, and the time of discharge from the practice. For reactions to SCIT, noting if there was a prior history of systemic reaction or asthma, the concentration of administered vials, volume administered, and if the vial was a new one are other essential pieces of information. It is recommended to grade the SCIT reaction according to the World Allergy Organization (WAO) criteria [6]. Other points to document include the patient's condition upon office discharge, instructions provided to the patient, and follow-up by an office provider on how the patient is faring after discharge. In cases where the reaction is severe, not responding to therapy, requiring more than one dose of epinephrine, or requiring IV fluids [2], EMS should be contacted. Providing a clinical vignette to the EMS providers along with documentation of medical therapies already rendered helps

Anaphylaxis Checklist and Flow Sheet

Name _____   Date _____

DOB _____   Allergens _____

Weight_____kg (lb/2.2) in children

History of Asthma: _____ Yes _____ No

If from immunotherapy, history of prior Systemic reaction: _____ Yes _____ No

Date/Time of Injection: _____   Date/Time of Reaction: _____

Vial color/#_____ Conc _____ Volume _____ New? Y ___ N ___ Local reaction_____

If not from immunotherapy, suspected trigger:_____

Signs & Symptoms: (circle pertinent findings)

> **Respiratory:** shortness of breath, chest tightness, wheezing, cough, stridor, itchy throat, hoarseness
>
> **Skin:** hives, swelling, itch, flushing
>
> **Eye/Nasal:** runny nose, red eyes, itchy eyes, congestion, sneezing
>
> **Vascular:** hypotension, chest discomfort, dizziness, syncope, headache
>
> **GI:** abdominal pain, nausea, vomiting, diarrhea
>
> **Other:** sweating, apprehension

Anaphylaxis Checklist

- ❖ Stop infusion, if applicable.
- ❖ Assess airway, breathing, circulation, and mentation.
- ❖ Obtain vital signs (BP, HR, O2 saturation).
- ❖ Lay patient flat. Pregnant patients in left lateral position. Pediatric patients in position of comfort.
- ❖ Give Epinephrine IM 1:1000. Adult: 0.3 to 0.5 mg. Pediatric: 0.01mg/kg up to max of 0.3 mg.
  - o 1st dose _____ cc IM   Time: _____
  - o 2nd dose _____ cc IM   Time: _____

Second dose of Epinephrine IM can be given if no response after 3–5 minutes. Max of 3 injections

- ❖ Administer O2 if hypotensive, SpO2 <95%, patient requires more than 1 epinephrine, beta agonists have been administered or preexisting risk factors for hypoxemia (facemask 8–10L/min).
- ❖ Obtain IV access (large bore IV). In adults, administer 1 L normal saline bolus if hypotensive. In pediatric patients administer 20–30ml/kg.
- ❖ If wheezing, shortness of breath, cough:
  - o Albuterol nebulizer
- ❖ Adjunct Medications:
  - o Benadryl 1 mg/kg PO or IM (up to 50 mg) _____ or Zyrtec 10 mg PO
  - o Solumedrol 2 mg/kg IM (up to 125 mg) or Prednisolone (15 mg/mL) or Prednisone PO _____
  - o Famotidine 20 mg/mL (up to 20 mg) _____
- ❖ Call 911. Y/N   Time Called: _____   Time Arrived: _____
- ❖ Call family member, emergency contact. Y/N   Time Called: _____
- ❖ Obtain tryptase level.

Patient Name_____   Date: _____

<u>ANAPHYLAXIS FLOW SHEET:</u>

Vital sign severy 5–15 minutes

Time	BP	HR	SpO2	PF	Interventions/Meds	Comments

Fig. 6.1 Sample anaphylaxis flow sheet

<u>ASSESSMENT AND PLAN</u>

Time of discharge from the office: _____ Anaphylaxis WAO Grade: _____
Condition upon release:
Vital signs stable: Y/N
All symptoms resolved: Y/N   If no, which symptoms remain_____
Patient instructions:
Signs, symptoms and treatment of anaphylaxis reviewed: Y/N
Anaphylaxis action plan provided: Y/N
Use of epinephrine autoinjector reviewed: Y/N
Risk of biphasic reactions reviewed: Y/N
Patient has epinephrine autoinjector: Y/N   If no, prescription sent to pharmacy: Y/N
Medications to take at home: _____

Dose Adjustment for IT? (Also document on IT sheet)
Recommendations_____

MD Signature: _____ RN Signature: _____
Follow-up call to patient
Date: _____   Time: _____
Comments:
_____

Fig. 6.1 (continued)

transition patients to the next healthcare setting. A sample office anaphylaxis document is available in the Joint Task Force practice parameters [5] and the adapted sheet the authors utilize in their office accompanies this chapter (Fig. 6.1).

Patient education on the signs and symptoms of anaphylaxis can begin the moment a procedure involving the risk is considered. Discussion of the risks and benefits should include a complete definition of anaphylaxis so that the patient has the ability to identify early signs and symptoms of a reaction. This education can be included during the informed consent process which should occur prior to starting any procedure with the risk of anaphylaxis [7]. Written consent, while not required for all procedures, may provide a framework for these conversations with both adults and minors. Consents should be framed in the context of the procedure (drug or food challenge, drug desensitization, SCIT, biologics for asthma, Ig replacement) being performed and its specific associated risks, including anaphylaxis. A written anaphylaxis action plan can be provided to the patient with instructions on anaphylaxis identification and management, including the administration of epinephrine [1].

Specific Procedure-Associated Risks

SCIT The office procedures most likely to be associated with anaphylaxis are administration of SCIT for aeroallergens and for venom. A trained physician, a qualified physician extender, or both should be present if SCIT is to be administered. SCIT should be administered in a facility with an emergency anaphylaxis kit or cart and personnel who are able to treat anaphylaxis [8]. Systemic reactions to SCIT range from mild to severe and fatal outcomes have been reported. Systemic reactions are estimated to occur with 0.1% of injection visits (or eight systemic reactions per 10,000 injection visits) and have been reported in 82–85% of practices [9]. Prior to 2002, fatal episodes were reported with a frequency of approximately three per year [10] but have been reported less frequently since that time [3, 9]. Poorly controlled asthma has been identified as a risk factor for life-threatening systemic reactions, and survey data suggests that increased screening for unstable asthma prior to SCIT administration may have contributed to the decline in fatal episodes [11].

Prevention of anaphylaxis is preferable to treatment, and careful selection of patients for procedures associated with risk may help decrease its frequency and severity. Screening for use of beta-blockers, ACE-Is in the case of venom IT, or significant pulmonary and cardiovascular comorbidities may identify patients who are not ideal candidates for SCIT or other at-risk procedures. Additionally, with SCIT, a standardized pre-injection questionnaire to review changes in medical condition, changes, or additions to medications and asthma control is recommended and may include peak flow measurement for asthmatics. Dosing errors have been reported as contributors to fatal and near-fatal anaphylaxis events [10, 12], and checkpoints to verify patient identity and appropriate dosing are important steps in each immunotherapy visit. Individually prepared and labelled vials allow for fewer distractions during mixing. Patient vials should be individually labelled with at least two patient identifiers (name, birthdate, assigned ID #, telephone #, and other patient-specific identifiers) as per the practice parameters which also provide specific instructions for dilution, nomenclature, and labelling of vials [8]. Less frequent mixing potentially reduces risks associated with different stock solution concentrations.

Cluster and rush immunotherapy have been associated with significantly more mild-to-moderate systemic reactions, and candidates for these procedures should be screened carefully [11]. Some data has suggested that premedication with antihistamines, prior to immunotherapy administration, decreased the frequency and severity of systemic reactions [13]. However this was not seen for cluster or conventional buildup in a prospective surveillance survey [11]. The immunotherapy practice parameters acknowledge that premedication prior to immunotherapy may lower risk, but there is no clear recommendation at this time [8]. A post-injection, in-office, 30-minute period of observation is generally regarded as standard of care [14]; however, there have been reports of anaphylaxis, including fatal anaphylaxis, occurring outside of this timeframe [8, 10]. While epinephrine auto-injectors are not required for all patients on SCIT, they may be considered for patients on SCIT or for any patient undergoing procedures with a risk of anaphylaxis [2, 8]. *Systemic reactions to SCIT should be classified according to the WAO grading system, which was recently modified* [48] (Fig. 6.2).

Oral food challenges A pooled estimate of anaphylaxis associated with oral food challenges (OFCs) was 2% in a multicenter analysis with a reaction rate of 14% for non-anaphylactic allergic reactions [15]; anaphylactic rates ranging between 11% and 14.7% [16, 17] have been seen in other studies of OFCs to various foods. Patient risk factors for severe reactions to OFCs include older age [17,

Modified World Allergy Organization Subcutaneous Immunotherapy Systemic Reaction Grading System				
Grade 1	Grade 2	Grade 3	Grade 4	Grade 5
Signs/Symptoms of 1 organ system:	Signs/Symptoms of 2 or more organ systems from Grade 1:			
Cutaneous: Urticaria and/or erythema-warmth and/or pruritus, other than localized at injection site And/or: Tingling or itch of the lips or Angioedema (not laryngeal) or **Upper Respiratory** Rhinitis And/or Throat clearing (Itchy Throat) And/or Cough (not related to bronchospasm) Or **Conjunctival** Erythema, itch or tearing or **Other** Nausea Metallic taste in mouth	**Cutaneous, Conjunctival, Upper respiratory, or Other nonspecific organ system**	**Lower Airway** Mild Bronchospasm And/or **Gastrointestinal** Abdominal cramps and/or vomiting/diarrhea **Other** Uterine cramps Any signs/symptoms from grade 1 would be included	**Lower Airway** Severe Bronchospasm And/or **Upper Airway** Laryngeal edema with stridor Any signs/symptoms from grade 1 or 3 would be included	**Lower or Upper Airway** Respiratory failure And/or **Cardiovascular** Collapse/hypotension And/or Loss of consciousness Any sign/symptom from grades 1, 3 or 4 would be included

Fig. 6.2 Modified WAO Subcutaneous IT Systemic Reaction Grading System. Key: Rhinitis: sneezing, rhinorrhea, nasal itch, and/or nasal congestion. Mild bronchospasm: cough, wheezing, shortness of breath that responds to treatment. Severe bronchospasm: not responding or worsening in spite of treatment. Hypotension defined: systolic BP <70 mm HG (in patients 1 month to 1 year of age). <70 mm Hg + [2x age] (in patients 1–10 years of age). <90 mm Hg (in patients 11–17 years of age). <90 mm Hg or >30% decrease in baseline (in adults patients). The final grade of the reaction is determined only when the event is over. Include the first symptom(s)/sign(s) and the time of onset after the injection. Note if epinephrine was administered by: (A) ≤5 min, (B) >5 min to less than or equal to ≤10 min, (C) >10 to 20 min, (D) >20 min. (Z) Epinephrine not administered. Final report: Grade 1–5; a–d or z; first symptom(s)/sign(s); time of onset of first symptom(s)/signs(s). (Table Adapted from the Cox et al. [48])

18] and possibly a history of an anaphylactic reaction [18] to the food in question though others have not seen this association [17]. Some studies have shown that high antigen-specific IgE level is itself a risk factor for an anaphylactic reaction during OFC [16], while others have indicated that there may be an association between the magnitude of the skin prick test and anaphylaxis [17]. While the risk of anaphylaxis during an OFC remains throughout the process, the risk does appear to increase with the amount of food ingested [17]. Continued assessment throughout the food challenge, including careful physical examination and assessment of vital signs prior to each subsequent stage, may allow clinicians to catch any early evidence of an allergic reaction [17].

As with other procedures associated with anaphylaxis, patients should undergo pre-challenge assessment since unstable or exacerbated atopic disease or concurrent upper respiratory infection might interfere with the challenge and increase the risk. Additionally, an elective food challenge should be deferred in patients with unstable comorbidities such as angina pectoris, cardiac disease, dysrhythmias, chronic lung disease, or pregnancy [19]. Obtaining vascular access should be considered prior to initiating an oral challenge in patients who would be deemed difficult cases. Additionally, ongoing medications should be reviewed, particularly cofactors such as aspirin and nonsteroidal anti-inflammatory drugs (NSAIDs) which have been noted to act as eliciting factors that might increase reactivity in susceptible patients [19]. Since beta-blockers may interfere with anaphylaxis treatment if epinephrine is required, clinicians need to weigh the risks and benefits of performing challenges in patients on these medications [19, 20].

Biologic Drugs Biologics administered parenterally are more likely to lead to hypersensitivity reactions. Some, like rituximab, have relatively high rates of systemic reactions with the first dose (5–10%) [21], while others more commonly used in the allergist's office like omalizumab have relatively low rates (0.09%) [22]. For omalizumab, an office wait time of 2 hours after the first three injections and 30 minutes thereafter is recommended [22]. Additionally, these patients should be prescribed an EAI to carry to and from omalizumab injection appointments [22]. For the newer biologics approved to treat asthma and atopic dermatitis, there is no standardized recommendation on office wait time.

Oral Drug Challenges Oral drug challenges (ODCs) are instrumental in the evaluation of a patient with a history of drug allergy ensuring that patients receive appropriate and often times cost-effective therapeutic options. ODCs are generally reserved for patients in whom the risk of immediate hypersensitivity is thought to be low, but our ability to use in vitro or in vivo testing to predict immediate-type reactivity is limited. Rates of systemic reactions during ODCs to medications (mostly antibiotics and NSAIDs) vary from 4.1% to 17.6% [23–26] with anaphylaxis reported in 3% of patients [23]. Proposed patient risk factors for reactive ODCs include females [23, 25] with multiple drug allergies [23]. Relative contraindications for ODCs are similar to OFCs and include pregnancy, acute illnesses, unstable asthma, or chronic systemic diseases [24].

Immunoglobulin While mild-to-moderate infusion reactions may occur in 5–15% of patients treated with IVIG, severe reactions, including anaphylaxis, occur in less than 1% of patients [27].

Vaccines The overall postvaccination rate of anaphylaxis was estimated in a review of children and adults vaccinated from 2009 to 2011 to be 1.31 cases of anaphylaxis per million vaccine doses, specifically, 1.35 cases per million doses of trivalent influenza vaccine and 2.48 cases per million doses of pneumococcal polysaccharide vaccine (PPSV23) [28].

Given that these reactions remain unpredictable, education for both patients and staff remains important safeguards [1].

Ongoing Training/Education

The Joint Task Force practice parameters recommend regular office anaphylaxis practice drills but do not give indications on how often to perform [5]. A survey conducted as part of quality improvement measure in allergy care queried if respondents performed mock anaphylaxis drills; of 33 respondents, 60% perform mock anaphylaxis drills in their offices, and 75% perform on a yearly basis [29]. Cardiopulmonary resuscitation certification for providers and nursing is also part of ongoing preparation for anaphylaxis [2, 7].

Introduction to Simulation for Anaphylaxis Training

The purpose of simulation is to replicate reality, and the term fidelity is used to describe the degree of realism [30]. Although its use is newer in healthcare, simulation has been used for many years in other fields including aviation and military training. The goal of simulation-based medical education is to provide the correct skills among healthcare providers to deal with real-life critical situations in a manner that does not compromise patients [30]. The simulator usually refers to a device that represents a simulated patient and interacts with the actions taken by the simulation participant [31]; simulators can be of low, medium, or high fidelity. Static mannequins are examples of low-fidelity simulators, while mannequins with mechanical movement may be of medium or high fidelity [30]. High-fidelity simulators are typically full-body mannequins that can communicate with participants (technician provides voice), have palpable pulses, and can display exam findings including cyanosis, rash, pupillary reflexes, or wheezing [30]. Simulation can be tailored to any level of physician education from those that are novices (medical students) to intermediate levels of education (residents and fellows in training) to experts (attendings) as well as other allied health disciplines (nursing, technicians, aides) [31]. The components of simulation include "immersion" into a clinical scenario/vignette, observation of the scenario, and feedback during a debriefing session afterward. The debriefing session explores what happened during the simulation and including how the participants felt and reinforces the educational goals or gaps addressed.

Studies have demonstrated that the hands-on practice offered by case simulations is more effective than standard classroom instruction for emergency situational training [32–34]. Simulations allow healthcare professionals to practice crises management, closed-loop communication, and teamwork skills to increase confidence in life-threatening emergencies [32] and allow for training of rare cases or unplanned events. They are the closest representation of a real-life emergency scenario without inflicting harm onto a real patient [32, 34], and direct observation during these simulations helps to uncover technical errors [35]. Simulations are used to assess performance of either an individual or a team [31]; they have been used in a wide variety of settings and for a wide variety of emergency training including cardiopulmonary arrest [36, 37], pediatric trauma and procedural techniques [38], and non-emergency training of surgical procedures [39].

Published simulation studies for anaphylaxis preparedness involve interdisciplinary team training with medical residents, fellows in training, attending faculty, and other healthcare professionals including nursing, mid-level providers, and emergency medical technicians ensuring that all members of a clinical team are prepared for this emergency. Radiologists have used simulations for the education of contrast-mediated anaphylaxis [40, 41], rheumatologists and oncologists for anaphylaxis in infusions centers [42, 43], and anesthesiologists for intraoperative anaphylaxis [44].

Anaphylaxis Simulation Use by Allergists/Immunologists

A program was developed by allergy and immunology and emergency medicine practitioners focusing on pediatric emergencies with four case-based scenarios utilizing a mixture of patient simulators (SIM Man 2G©, SIM Baby 1G© Laerdal Medical) and standardized patients [45]. The first case involved an 18-month-old infant presenting acutely to the office due to peanut anaphylaxis, and the second case involved anaphylaxis in the office post a dose of venom immunotherapy. An algorithm was followed based on the actions of the participants; if milestones were not reached, then the high-fidelity simulator would display a change in vitals/physical exam. In this study, there were 26 participants including a mixture of physicians, nurses, office administrators, and respiratory therapists from both hospital- and community-based allergy clinics. Three independent reviewers evaluated team performance in terms of role clarity, communication, teamwork, situational awareness, and scenario-specific skills. Both the community-based allergy and the hospital-based allergy clinics showed improvement in total team competency scores from baseline to each subsequent scenario in a mixed model analysis ($p < 0.01$). Ten to 12 months later, an unannounced simulation (repeat of case 1) was performed in the allergy (in situ) clinics. Taken together, both the hospital-based and community-based allergy clinics demonstrated significant statistical improvement at this time point in comparison to their initial case suggesting a sustained change in knowledge and skills almost 1 year later.

Anaphylaxis Simulation Use by Other Specialists

In another article, a total of 72 workshop participants (divided in 14 groups) that included nurses, mid-level healthcare professionals (nurse practitioners, physician assistants), and physicians in the Division of Hematology and Oncology determined whether participants recognized and treated anaphylaxis appropriately via a high-fidelity patient simulator [42]. The simulation involved SimMan 3G© (Laerdal Medical) that developed wheezing, urticaria, and hypotension while receiving his 7th dose of carboplatin. A scenario algorithm was implemented whereby SimMan's clinical condition deteriorated as the case progressed without epinephrine administration. Eight of the 14 groups (57%) administered an EAI prior to the use of antihistamines and or systemic corticosteroids (CS). Knowledge gaps addressed for the use of medications besides epinephrine included participant's beliefs: that epinephrine should be used only if symptoms were refractory to antihistamines and corticosteroids; that treating with epinephrine would label patients as being chemotherapy allergic and delay future infusions; that epinephrine should not be administered without the presence of cutaneous symptoms (these participants failed to appreciate the rash underneath the mannequin's gown); and that epinephrine should not be administered in a patient with an unknown cardiac history. These beliefs emphasize the continued barriers that must be addressed to optimize the medical management of anaphylaxis, namely, epinephrine as first-line therapy.

Rheumatology fellows and recent graduates ($n = 18$) participated in simulation curriculum case involving a patient in the infusion center experiencing an acute infusion reaction to a biologic [43]. Their performance was evaluated by a predetermined checklist that graded the participants on how they obtained a relevant history and managed an infusion reaction. All participants discontinued the infusion after recognizing anaphylaxis, and most activated an emergency response system. However, epinephrine was administered by only 56% ($n = 10$). Adjunct medications that were administered included steroids by 72% ($n = 13$), and 56% ($n = 10$) ordered antihistamines. Pre-participation fellow surveys indicated that participants were uncomfortable managing an acute infusion reaction (10/18) or felt that they had poor knowledge to manage an acute infusion reaction (11/18). Post this activity, all (18/18) felt that the training was worth their time and effort and their knowledge was improved. Taken together, these two studies demonstrate that epinephrine is still not first-line therapy even when anaphylaxis is recognized and addressing knowledge gaps for its administration remains essential.

A cohort study was used to assess the recognition and management of anaphylaxis with and without hypotension in a standardized scenario using a patient simulator (MegaCode Kid© Laerdal Medical) [46]. The primary outcome measure was the administration of adrenaline in emergency department junior staff. The group was divided into two: group 1 ($n = 28$) completing a standard scenario of a child with anaphylaxis (generalized urticaria, shortness of breath, and wheeze) including hypotension, while group 2 ($n = 28$) completed the same standard anaphylaxis scenario, but the patient was normotensive. A total of 28 (50%) participants administered parenteral adrenaline; significantly more participants from group 1 (21/28; 75%) gave parenteral adrenaline compared with group 2 (normotensive patient) (7/28; 25%) ($P < 0.001$). Despite guideline definition of anaphylaxis [5] and the recommendation to treat early, the presence of hypotension (shock) still appears to be a strong motivator for epinephrine administration. Post-simulation, all participants agreed or strongly agreed that the participation had improved their knowledge, that they would recommend the program to others, and that they enjoyed this educational tool.

Anaphylaxis Simulation Use by EMS

Two- and four-person emergency medical services crews from eight geographically diverse agencies in Michigan participated in a 20-minute simulation of a 5-year-old child with an anaphylactic reaction to a bee sting [47]. The high-fidelity simulator (Pediatric 5-Year-Old Hal Abacus Dx©) had acute onset of urticaria, wheezing, shortness of breath, and hypotension (>30% decrease in systolic blood pressure). A total of 142 EMTs, licensed emergency medicine specialists, and paramedics participated in 62 simulation sessions. The participants responded to the simulated emergency inside the mobile simulation unit with equipment, supplies, and drugs from their own ambulances. Epinephrine was administered in 95% of scenarios ($n = 59/62$), but only 46% ($n = 27/59$) gave the correct dose in the appropriate route. Twelve crews (20%) gave a dose that was ≥5 times the correct dose, and eight crews (14%) bolused epinephrine intravenously instead. Reasons for medication errors included weight estimation errors, faulty recall of medication doses, calculation errors, dose estimation and communication errors. As advocates for our specialty, educational efforts may need to extend to our colleagues in the community including first responders.

Although anaphylaxis simulation studies to date have small numbers of participants, variable clinical scenarios, and different outcome measures, it appears that there is a positive effect in education. In some circumstances, that effect appears maintained, but not all studies have queried participants at later dates to confirm a definitive change in knowledge, outcomes, or behaviors post participation. Simulation is well accepted by participants and can be adapted to various levels of training; teams can be mixed with multiple disciplines and/or specialties. Simulation is also the closest "real-life" educational activity that providers can participate in without placing patients at risk or breaking confidentiality. However regardless of the type of education, it is apparent that providing continued education on the identification and management of anaphylaxis is needed across different specialties and disciplines as the range of epinephrine administration in the above-quoted studies ranged from a low of 25% in patients without hypotension [46] to a high of 95% (although only 46% gave the correct dose in that study) [47]. The authors utilize anaphylaxis simulation as continued preparedness for all our office staff including front desk, nursing, fellows in training, mid-level providers, and attendings; we also advocate for continued quality improvement for our institution and have used anaphylaxis simulations in training with the Hematology/Oncology [42] Division and the Internal Medicine Division [49].

References

1. Lieberman P, Nicklas RA, Randolph C, Oppenheimer J, Bernstein D, Bernstein J, et al. Anaphylaxis--a practice parameter update 2015. Ann Allergy Asthma Immunol. 2015;115(5):341–84.
2. Wallace DV. Anaphylaxis in the allergist's office: preparing your office and staff for medical emergencies. Allergy Asthma Proc. 2013;34(2):120–31.

3. Amin HS, Liss GM, Bernstein DI. Evaluation of near-fatal reactions to allergen immunotherapy injections. J Allergy Clin Immunol. 2006;117(1):169–75.
4. Sampson HA, Mendelson L, Rosen JP. Fatal and near-fatal anaphylactic reactions to food in children and adolescents. N Engl J Med. 1992;327(6):380–4.
5. Lieberman P, Nicklas RA, Oppenheimer J, Kemp SF, Lang DM, Bernstein DI, et al. The diagnosis and management of anaphylaxis practice parameter: 2010 update. J Allergy Clin Immunol. 2010;126(3):477–80. e1–42.
6. Cox L, Larenas-Linnemann D, Lockey RF, Passalacqua G. Speaking the same language: The World Allergy Organization subcutaneous immunotherapy systemic reaction grading system. J Allergy Clin Immunol. 2010;125(3):569–74, 74 e1–74 e7.
7. Cingi C, Wallace D, Bayar Muluk N, Ebisawa M, Castells M, Sahin E, et al. Managing anaphylaxis in the office setting. Am J Rhinol Allergy. 2016;30(4):118–23.
8. Cox L, Nelson H, Lockey R, Calabria C, Chacko T, Finegold I, et al. Allergen immunotherapy: a practice parameter third update. J Allergy Clin Immunol. 2011;127(1 Suppl):S1–55.
9. Epstein TG, Liss GM, Murphy-Berendts K, Bernstein DI. AAAAI/ACAAI surveillance study of subcutaneous immunotherapy, years 2008-2012: an update on fatal and nonfatal systemic allergic reactions. J Allergy Clin Immunol Pract. 2014;2(2):161–7.
10. Bernstein DI, Wanner M, Borish L, Liss GM, Immunotherapy Committee AAoAA, Immunology. Twelve-year survey of fatal reactions to allergen injections and skin testing: 1990-2001. J Allergy Clin Immunol. 2004;113(6):1129–36.
11. Epstein TG, Liss GM, Murphy-Berendts K, Bernstein DI. AAAAI and ACAAI surveillance study of subcutaneous immunotherapy, Year 3: what practices modify the risk of systemic reactions? Ann Allergy Asthma Immunol. 2013;110(4):274–8, 8 e1.
12. Lockey RF, Benedict LM, Turkeltaub PC, Bukantz SC. Fatalities from immunotherapy (IT) and skin testing (ST). J Allergy Clin Immunol. 1987;79(4):660–77.
13. Ohashi Y, Nakai Y, Murata K. Effect of pretreatment with fexofenadine on the safety of immunotherapy in patients with allergic rhinitis. Ann Allergy Asthma Immunol. 2006;96(4):600–5.
14. Cox L, Esch RE, Corbett M, Hankin C, Nelson M, Plunkett G. Allergen immunotherapy practice in the United States: guidelines, measures, and outcomes. Ann Allergy Asthma Immunol. 2011;107(4):289–99; quiz 300.
15. Akuete K, Guffey D, Israelsen RB, Broyles JM, Higgins LJ, Green TD, et al. Multicenter prevalence of anaphylaxis in clinic-based oral food challenges. Ann Allergy Asthma Immunol. 2017;119(4):339–48. e1.
16. Yanagida N, Sato S, Takahashi K, Nagakura KI, Asaumi T, Ogura K, et al. Increasing specific immunoglobulin E levels correlate with the risk of anaphylaxis during an oral food challenge. Pediatr Allergy Immunol. 2018;29(4):417–24.
17. Arkwright PD, MacMahon J, Koplin J, Rajput S, Cross S, Fitzsimons R, et al. Severity and threshold of peanut reactivity during hospital-based open oral food challenges: an international multicenter survey. Pediatr Allergy Immunol. 2018;29(7):754–61.
18. Yanagida N, Sato S, Asaumi T, Ogura K, Ebisawa M. Risk factors for severe reactions during double-blind placebo-controlled food challenges. Int Arch Allergy Immunol. 2017;172(3):173–82.
19. Sampson HA, Gerth van Wijk R, Bindslev-Jensen C, Sicherer S, Teuber SS, Burks AW, et al. Standardizing double-blind, placebo-controlled oral food challenges: American Academy of Allergy, Asthma & Immunology-European Academy of Allergy and Clinical Immunology PRACTALL consensus report. J Allergy Clin Immunol. 2012;130(6):1260–74.
20. Nowak-Wegrzyn A, Assa'ad AH, Bahna SL, Bock SA, Sicherer SH, Teuber SS, et al. Work group report: oral food challenge testing. J Allergy Clin Immunol. 2009;123(6 Suppl):S365–83.
21. Grillo-Lopez AJ, White CA, Dallaire BK, Varns CL, Shen CD, Wei A, et al. Rituximab: the first monoclonal antibody approved for the treatment of lymphoma. Curr Pharm Biotechnol. 2000;1(1):1–9.
22. Cox L, Platts-Mills TA, Finegold I, Schwartz LB, Simons FE, Wallace DV, et al. American Academy of Allergy, Asthma & Immunology/American College of Allergy, Asthma and

Immunology Joint Task Force Report on omalizumab-associated anaphylaxis. J Allergy Clin Immunol. 2007;120(6):1373–7.

23. Mawhirt SL, Fonacier LS, Calixte R, Davis-Lorton M, Aquino MR. Skin testing and drug challenge outcomes in antibiotic-allergic patients with immediate-type hypersensitivity. Ann Allergy Asthma Immunol. 2017;118(1):73–9.

24. Aun MV, Bisaccioni C, Garro LS, Rodrigues AT, Tanno LK, Ensina LF, et al. Outcomes and safety of drug provocation tests. Allergy Asthma Proc. 2011;32(4):301–6.

25. Iammatteo M, Blumenthal KG, Saff R, Long AA, Banerji A. Safety and outcomes of test doses for the evaluation of adverse drug reactions: a 5-year retrospective review. J Allergy Clin Immunol Pract. 2014;2(6):768–74.

26. Messaad D, Sahla H, Benahmed S, Godard P, Bousquet J, Demoly P. Drug provocation tests in patients with a history suggesting an immediate drug hypersensitivity reaction. Ann Intern Med. 2004;140(12):1001–6.

27. Brennan VM, Salome-Bentley NJ, Chapel HM, Immunology NS. Prospective audit of adverse reactions occurring in 459 primary antibody-deficient patients receiving intravenous immunoglobulin. Clin Exp Immunol. 2003;133(2):247–51.

28. McNeil MM, Weintraub ES, Duffy J, Sukumaran L, Jacobsen SJ, Klein NP, et al. Risk of anaphylaxis after vaccination in children and adults. J Allergy Clin Immunol. 2016;137(3):868–78.

29. Lee S, Stachler RJ, Ferguson BJ. Defining quality metrics and improving safety and outcome in allergy care. Int Forum Allergy Rhinol. 2014;4(4):284–91.

30. Datta R, Upadhyay K, Jaideep C. Simulation and its role in medical education. Med J Armed Forces India. 2012;68(2):167–72.

31. Gaba DM. The future vision of simulation in healthcare. Simul Healthc. 2007;2(2):126–35.

32. Lighthall GK, Barr J. The use of clinical simulation systems to train critical care physicians. J Intensive Care Med. 2007;22(5):257–69.

33. Maddry JK, Varney SM, Sessions D, Heard K, Thaxton RE, Ganem VJ, et al. A comparison of simulation-based education versus lecture-based instruction for toxicology training in emergency medicine residents. J Med Toxicol. 2014;10(4):364–8.

34. Ten Eyck RP, Tews M, Ballester JM. Improved medical student satisfaction and test performance with a simulation-based emergency medicine curriculum: a randomized controlled trial. Ann Emerg Med. 2009;54(5):684–91.

35. Ziv A, Ben-David S, Ziv M. Simulation based medical education: an opportunity to learn from errors. Med Teach. 2005;27(3):193–9.

36. Hunziker S, Buhlmann C, Tschan F, Balestra G, Legeret C, Schumacher C, et al. Brief leadership instructions improve cardiopulmonary resuscitation in a high-fidelity simulation: a randomized controlled trial. Crit Care Med. 2010;38(4):1086–91.

37. Wayne DB, Didwania A, Feinglass J, Fudala MJ, Barsuk JH, McGaghie WC. Simulation-based education improves quality of care during cardiac arrest team responses at an academic teaching hospital: a case-control study. Chest. 2008;133(1):56–61.

38. Weinberg ER, Auerbach MA, Shah NB. The use of simulation for pediatric training and assessment. Curr Opin Pediatr. 2009;21(3):282–7.

39. Zendejas B, Cook DA, Bingener J, Huebner M, Dunn WF, Sarr MG, et al. Simulation-based mastery learning improves patient outcomes in laparoscopic inguinal hernia repair: a randomized controlled trial. Ann Surg. 2011;254(3):502–9; discussion 9-11.

40. Pfeifer K, Staib L, Arango J, Kirsch J, Arici M, Kappus L, et al. High-fidelity contrast reaction simulation training: performance comparison of faculty, fellows, and residents. J Am Coll Radiol. 2016;13(1):81–7.

41. Niell BL, Kattapuram T, Halpern EF, Salazar GM, Penzias A, Bonk SS, et al. Prospective analysis of an interprofessional team training program using high-fidelity simulation of contrast reactions. AJR Am J Roentgenol. 2015;204(6):W670–6.

42. Chong M, Pasqua D, Kutzin J, Davis-Lorton M, Fonacier L, Aquino M. Educational and process improvements after a simulation-based anaphylaxis simulation workshop. Ann Allergy Asthma Immunol. 2016;117(4):432–3.

43. Weiner JJ, Eudy AM, Criscione-Schreiber LG. How well do rheumatology fellows manage acute infusion reactions? A pilot curricular intervention. Arthritis Care Res (Hoboken). 2018;70(6):931–7.
44. Johnston EB, King C, Sloane PA, Cox JW, Youngblood AQ, Lynn Zinkan J, et al. Pediatric anaphylaxis in the operating room for anesthesia residents: a simulation study. Paediatr Anaesth. 2017;27(2):205–10.
45. Kennedy JL, Jones SM, Porter N, White ML, Gephardt G, Hill T, et al. High-fidelity hybrid simulation of allergic emergencies demonstrates improved preparedness for office emergencies in pediatric allergy clinics. J Allergy Clin Immunol Pract. 2013;1(6):608–17. e1–14.
46. O'Leary FM, Hokin B, Enright K, Campbell DE. Treatment of a simulated child with anaphylaxis: an in situ two-arm study. J Paediatr Child Health. 2013;49(7):541–7.
47. Lammers R, Willoughby-Byrwa M, Fales W. Medication errors in prehospital management of simulated pediatric anaphylaxis. Prehosp Emerg Care. 2014;18(2):295–304.
48. Cox LS, Sanchez-Borges M, Lockey RF. World Allergy Organization systemic allergic reaction grading system: is a modification needed? J Allergy Clin Immunol Pract. 2017;5(I):58–62.
49. Stephanie L. Mawhirt DO, Luz Fonacier MD, Marcella R. Aquino, MD. Utilization of high-fidelity simulation for medical student and resident education of allergicimmunologic emergencies. Ann Allergy Asthma Immunol. 2019;122(5):513–21. (PMID: 30802501).

Masqueraders of Anaphylaxis

Julia E. M. Upton

Anaphylaxis is a clinically defined condition [1, 2], and there can be instances where there are difficulties determining whether a person has experienced anaphylaxis or whether it is a different disorder.

This chapter will address the differential diagnosis of anaphylaxis: conditions which can mimic or masquerade as anaphylaxis. The disorders will be considered in terms of their dominant symptoms (Table 7.1).

This chapter will not elaborate on unusual underlying *causes* of anaphylaxis (Table 7.2) which are sometimes classified under the differential diagnosis of anaphylaxis such as anaphylaxis from histamine-release syndromes [3] including from the hydatid cyst of *Echinococcus granulosus* [4], from anisakiasis [5, 6], or from basophilic leukemia [7] and from the treatment of acute promyelocytic leukemia with tretinoin [8]. It will also not elaborate on temporary causes of anaphylaxis in a non-allergic person as can be seen in passive transfer of IgE from blood donors [9, 10].

Mastocytosis [11] deserves special mention because it is an underlying cause of anaphylaxis, but it is also commonly considered in the differential diagnosis of anaphylaxis [3, 12–15]. It is important to consider mastocytosis in anaphylaxis to hymenoptera [12] as well as in unexplained anaphylaxis, flushing, osteoporosis, gastrointestinal ulcerative disease, or chronic abdominal cramping [16]. Mast cell activation syndromes [17] can also present as anaphylaxis [18]. A normal tryptase does not rule out a clonal mast cell disorder, and a high level of suspicion of mast cell disease is required [16].

J. E. M. Upton (✉)
Division of Immunology and Allergy, Hospital for Sick Children, Toronto, ON, Canada

Department of Paediatrics, University of Toronto, Toronto, ON, Canada
e-mail: Julia.upton@sickkids.ca

© Springer Nature Switzerland AG 2020
A. K. Ellis (ed.), *Anaphylaxis*, https://doi.org/10.1007/978-3-030-43205-8_7

Table 7.1 Mimickers of anaphylaxis by the dominant symptom

Predominantly skin symptoms
  Urticaria syndromes
  Angioedema
    Hereditary
    Acquired
    Idiopathic
  Flushing
    Rosacea
    Emotional
    Hormonal flushing (menopause, hypoandrogen state)
    Neuroendocrine tumors (including carcinoid, pheochromocytoma, VIPoma
    Other malignancies such as renal cell carcinoma
    Drug/infusion associated (e.g., red man syndrome from vancomycin, infusion reactions from chemotherapy)
    Toxin associated (e.g., scombroidosis, organophosphates)
    Autonomic dysregulation
Predominantly respiratory symptoms
  Asthma
  Vocal cord paralysis
  Aspiration/foreign body
Loss of consciousness/syncope
  Stroke/transient ischemic attack
  Syncope
    Reflex (vasovagal)
    Orthostatic
    Cardiovascular
  Seizures
Shock
  Distributive
  Hypovolemic
  Cardiogenic
Predominantly gastrointestinal symptoms
  Neuroendocrine tumors
  Abdominal migraine/cyclical vomiting
Postprandial
  Swallowing syncope
  Food protein-induced enterocolitis (FPIES)
  Aspiration/foreign body
  Hypoglycemia
  Pollen-food syndrome
  Food poisoning
  Toxic effects such as ackee fruit, scombroidosis (fish)
Non-organic

Predominantly Skin Symptoms

Urticaria

One of the challenges the allergist faces is to determine if the patient experienced anaphylaxis or only cutaneous-limited symptoms. Cutaneous symptoms occur in approximately 90% of anaphylactic events [3]. Urticaria is defined as a skin

Table 7.2 Causes of endogenous histamine release leading to anaphylaxis

Mastocytosis
Mast cell activation syndromes
Parasitic disease (*Echinococcus granulosus*, anisakiasis)
Basophilic leukemia
Acute promyelocytic leukemia treated with tretinoin

condition of wheals, angioedema, or both. Urticaria may have been diagnosed or treated as anaphylaxis by emergency services or by the patient.

The distinction between urticaria syndromes and anaphylaxis relies on describing the urticarial lesions in the absence of other systemic features of anaphylaxis.

Urticaria lesions have three characteristics:

1. A central swelling of variable size, almost invariably surrounded by reflex erythema.
2. Symptoms of itching or sometimes burning.
3. The skin where the urticaria was located returns to normal within 30 minutes to 24 hours [19].

The urticarial syndromes include acute urticaria lasting less than 6 weeks and chronic urticaria lasting more than 6 weeks. Chronic urticaria can be subdivided into chronic spontaneous urticaria (CSU) and inducible urticaria from physical triggers such as cold, delayed pressure, heat, water, vibration, cholinergic contact, sunlight, or dermatographism [19]. There are additionally multiple mimickers of urticaria [20, 21] including hereditary autoinflammatory syndromes such as cryopyrin-associated periodic syndromes and familial cold autoinflammatory syndrome and acquired autoinflammatory syndromes of Schnitzler syndrome and others. These urticaria mimickers are suspected on clinical grounds when the skin lesions last more than 24 hours, or if they leave discoloration, or if there are additional symptoms such as a family history of similar lesions, fever, joint/bone pain, or deafness. Abnormal laboratory results of an elevated erythrocyte sedimentation rate and abnormal complete blood count with differential also lead to further investigation of urticaria.

Sometimes the distinction between urticaria and anaphylaxis is blurred. In some urticarial syndromes, a low threshold of suspicion of concomitant anaphylaxis must be maintained. The cold- and cholinergic-inducible urticaria can progress to anaphylaxis [22]. Furthermore, urticaria may have been diagnosed when a person has actually experienced anaphylaxis. In a recent study of 1051 pediatric patients with urticaria at a university hospital emergency department, 37 were found to be anaphylaxis by clinical criteria [23].

Angioedema

Angioedema can accompany anaphylaxis but is also a mimicker of anaphylaxis [24]. In addition to the angioedema seen in some urticarial syndromes such as CSU discussed above, syndromes with predominant angioedema can be mimickers of anaphylaxis. The disorders of C1 esterase, hereditary angioedema (HAE) type 1 and 2 [25, 26], as well as acquired angioedema (AAE) [27] can present as life-threatening swelling.

Medications are a very important cause of isolated angioedema, with the best-described angiotensin-converting enzyme inhibitors [28, 29] as well as NSAIDs [29, 30].

There is increasing recognition of other pathways which can cause angioedema syndromes which do not involve C1 esterase [31, 32].

There are other causes of swelling which may be referred to an allergist as angioedema and be mistaken for an allergic cause. Erythropoietic protoporphyria can present with angioedema and rashes after sun exposure although the relationship to the solar exposure is not always immediately apparent to the patient [33]. Serum-free protoporphyrin is diagnostic.

The distinction of angioedema syndromes from anaphylaxis requires the lack of other systems. This distinction can be difficult because angioedema can cause respiratory symptoms of cough and dyspnea and gastrointestinal symptoms such as nausea and pain from intestinal wall swelling. Although classically the C1 esterase-medicated angioedema does not have a rash, they can have erythema marginatum, an erythematous serpiginous rash [25]. Many allergists maintain a low threshold to consider an angioedema syndrome in the differential diagnosis of anaphylaxis and vice versa.

The classification of angioedema considers the clinical presentation (urticaria or no urticaria), the pattern of inheritance, the pathophysiology, and the response to therapy [34, 35]. Laboratory analysis of angioedema involves the interrogation of the C1 esterase pathway with C4, C1 esterase inhibitor level and function, as well as C1q if AAE is suspected [36]. More specialized tests for less common angioedema syndromes, including factor XII, are also available [36].

Flushing Syndromes

Flushing syndromes are a classic mimicker of anaphylaxis because flushing occurs in approximately 50% of anaphylactic events [3]. Flushing can be separated into wet or dry [37, 38] based on whether they are accompanied by perspiration/diaphoresis. Flushing syndromes may also be focussed on those with malignant causes [39] or with or without gastrointestinal complaints [40, 41]. The episodic flushing syndromes can mimic anaphylaxis, and because many of the causative underlying diseases are rare, they may not be initially considered.

Wet Flushing

The wet flushing syndromes are autonomic nervous system mediated. Wet flushing can be from exogenous or endogenous causes. Simple blushing from an emotional cause is one of the most common endogenous causes. Other common causes are from thermoregulation in heat or fever [42].

Hormonal causes of wet flushing include menopausal symptoms in women or a hypo-androgenic state in men and other endocrinological disorders such as hyperthyroidism [42].

Pheochromocytoma is a rare but well-described cause of wet flushing. Pheochromocytoma is a neuroendocrine tumor which develops from the chromaffin cells and releases epinephrine, norepinephrine, and dopamine [43]. Less than half of pheochromocytoma patients will have the classic triad of headache, palpitations, and diaphoresis. A high level of suspicion of pheochromocytoma is required because it is so rare and it can be deadly if not diagnosed. Total fractionated urine metanephrines (metadrenalines) or plasma-free metanephrines should be used as an initial biochemical screen for PPGL [44].

There are multiple autonomic nervous system disorders which present with wet flushing including auriculotemporal syndrome and diencephalic autonomic epilepsy. Other neurological conditions can also be accompanied by autonomic dysregulation including Parkinson's disease, migraine, multiple sclerosis, trigeminal nerve damage, Horner syndrome, autonomic hyperreflexia, orthostatic hypotension, and postural orthostatic tachycardia syndrome (POTS) [39, 42, 45].

Paroxysmal extreme pain disorder is a rare sodium channelopathy of monogenic cause (SCN9A) which was previously referred to as familial rectal pain syndrome and presents with flushing and pain in the rectal and mouth areas [46]. The flushing can be in a harlequin pattern, and there can be syncopal events due to the autonomic dysfunction.

Mesenteric traction syndrome is a syndrome of flushing, tachycardia, and arterial hypotension due to mast cell mediator release from gut manipulation during surgery [47] and can mimic intraoperative anaphylaxis.

Medications and toxins can be exogenous causes of wet flushing, an example of which is serotonin reuptake inhibitors [38]. Most medications are classified under dry flushing. Organophosphate poisoning is a known cause of wet flushing which causes nausea, vomiting, abdominal pain, and copious secretions and can lead to coma and seizures [48]. Exposure to organophosphates at these toxic levels would typically require occupational exposure.

Dry Flushing

The dry flushing syndromes are vasodilator mediated. Dry flushing can be further separated into endogenous and exogenous causes.

The endogenous causes of dry flushing can be divided into malignant and nonmalignant causes. Nonmalignant causes of wet flushing [45] include rosacea and emotional flushing. Less common causes are dumping syndrome, benign mast cell disorders, sarcoid, and mitral stenosis.

Endogenous neoplastic/malignant causes include neuroendocrine tumors (NET) including "carcinoid" tumors producing the carcinoid syndrome [49]. The main clinical features of carcinoid syndrome are flushing and diarrhea, and patients may also have abdominal pain and even wheezing. The symptoms will differ depending on the tumor locations, with the classic carcinoid syndrome associated with tumors in the mid-gut. It should be noted that since 2000, the World Health Organization advocates for the term carcinoid as it relates to the tumor to be replaced with the term NET. The most useful screening test is 24-hour urine for 5-HIAA. Other NETs which can cause flushing include pancreatic NETs releasing VIP, neurotensin, insulin, glucagon, prostaglandin, and other hormones [37].

Medullary carcinoma of the thyroid is a rare cancer which releases calcitonin [50] and can also secrete histamine and other chemicals. These tumors can cause flushing, pruritus, and diarrhea, although diarrhea is the most common symptom. The main risk factors are inherited multiple endocrine neoplasia and older age [51]. Serum calcitonin is usually elevated. It does not typically affect thyroid-stimulating hormone levels.

Multiple other rare malignant causes of flushing have been described including polyradiculoneuropathy, organomegaly, endocrinopathy, renal cell carcinoma, monoclonal plasma cell disorder (POEMS syndrome), bronchogenic carcinoma, malignant histiocytoma, malignant neuroblastoma, malignant ganglioglioma, Leigh syndrome, and superior vena cava syndrome [39, 42].

Exogenous causes of dry flushing include many medications such as niacin, alcohol, calcium channel blockers, vancomycin, NSAIDs, narcotics, psychiatric medications [42], and chemotherapy infusions [52, 53]. Flushing requires a detailed medication history of all prescribed and over-the-counter medications.

Additional exogenous causes of flushing can be found in foods. Scombroidosis is a toxic exogenous cause of flushing from spoiled histidine-containing fish such as tuna, mackerel, and swordfish [54].

The diversity of the flushing syndromes requires a comprehensive approach to their evaluation. One recommended approach to the diagnosis of flushing considers the serious causes first. In this approach, if the history and physical exam have not revealed a diagnosis, laboratory tests are initially directed to serious causes [42] including pheochromocytoma, carcinoid, and mastocytosis (serum tryptase). If those evaluations have not suggested the cause, then follow with investigating for renal cell carcinoma (urinalysis for hematuria), pancreatic cell carcinoma (VIP level), and medullary thyroid carcinoma (calcitonin and thyroid imaging), as well as a referral to an allergist and endocrinologist.

Another initial approach suggested for flushing is to distinguish between wet and dry. If wet, consider hypogonadism. If no evidence of hypogonadism, consider pheochromocytoma. If dry, first consider if medications is the cause. If no medications appear to be causative, then consider neuroendocrine tumor, pheochromocytoma, mastocytosis, VIPoma, and medullary thyroid carcinoma, refer to an allergist. There is also a consideration of a trial of octreotide treatment [38].

Allergists evaluating a patient for flushing may pay special attention to anaphylaxis as well as mastocytosis (tryptase and c-kit), urticaria, and angioedema (c1 esterase inhibitor level and function, C4, and C1q) as potential causes of the flushing [38, 42].

Predominantly Respiratory Symptoms

Thus far this chapter has considered anaphylaxis mimics where the skin is the dominant factor (urticaria, angioedema, and flushing). However, anaphylaxis does not always have skin symptoms. It is estimated that approximately 10% of anaphylaxis presentations do not include urticaria [3]. When anaphylaxis occurs without urticaria, it becomes harder to recognize, and anaphylaxis without skin symptoms may be a sign of more severe reactions with a higher fatality rate [55].

Respiratory symptoms of dyspnea and wheeze are common in anaphylaxis, occurring at a rate of approximately 60% [3], and therefore there are respiratory mimics of anaphylaxis.

Asthma

Asthma is an obstructive lung disease characterized by wheezing, chest tightness, and shortness of breath, and progress to respiratory failure [56]. Both asthma and anaphylaxis can present with these same respiratory symptoms. Anaphylaxis will have another system involved, but these symptoms may not be apparent initially.

Asthma symptoms can mimic those of anaphylaxis and vice versa. Patients who have both asthma and food allergies can find it difficult to know if they are having an asthma exacerbation or anaphylaxis [57]. A low threshold to use epinephrine auto-injectors in asthmatic symptoms can be advised in patients with known concurrent asthma [58]. In a study of 105 adults admitted to an intensive care unit in New York for asthma, 7/88 (8.0%) met diagnostic criteria for anaphylaxis, and 3/88 (3.4%) were deemed highly likely to have had anaphylaxis [59] using the 2011 World Allergy Organization (WAO) criteria [60]. In this retrospective study, only one of these seven patients was prescribed epinephrine auto-injector and referred to an allergist.

Other acute respiratory events which can masquerade as asthma and therefore masquerade as anaphylaxis can include epiglottitis, chronic obstructive pulmonary disease, congestive heart failure, gastrointestinal reflux, pneumothorax, central airway obstruction, and pulmonary embolism [56].

Wheezing in infancy is a special circumstance because the differential diagnosis is very broad including asthma as well as cardiac disease, anatomical causes such as vascular ring, tracheomalacia, multiple congenital diseases of the lungs, infections such as bronchiolitis or epiglottitis, and foreign body aspiration [61].

Vocal Cord Dysfunction

Vocal cord dysfunction (VCD) [62] is recognized to mimic asthma and can also mimic anaphylaxis [63, 64]. VCD is characterized by paradoxical movement of the vocal cords and presents with respiratory symptoms of dyspnea, cough, and wheeze. VCD is typically triggered by emotional distress. The diagnosis can be made by characteristic findings on spirometry although direct visualization of the cords may be required by otolaryngology.

Aspiration

Acute foreign body aspiration can also mimic anaphylaxis and vice versa, especially when it occurs in the setting of eating [65].

Collapse/Altered or Loss of Consciousness

In anaphylaxis, the systemic vasodilation can cause significant hypotension with decreased blood flow to the brain and subsequent altered levels of consciousness or even collapse. Dizziness, hypotension, and syncope are estimated to occur in 35% of anaphylactic events [3]. Therefore, there are multiple disorders which can mimic the cardiovascular and neurological symptoms and signs of anaphylaxis.

Transient Loss of Consciousness

Anaphylaxis can rarely present as a transient loss of consciousness with no skin symptoms, followed by confusion and neurological signs, and incite the differential diagnosis of stroke or transient ischemic attack [66]. A careful history of precipitating factors may reveal a preceding trigger for anaphylaxis, such as a hymenoptera sting, in some cases of TLC [67]. To further complicate matters, the hypoperfusion of anaphylaxis can cause ischemic and thromboembolic strokes [68–70].

A transient loss of consciousness is typically caused by, in order of frequency, syncope, epileptic seizures, psychogenic transient loss of consciousness, and a miscellaneous group of rare causes [71–74].

Syncope

Syncope [67, 75–80] has a large differential diagnosis. The three main groups of syncope are reflex (vasovagal), orthostatic, and cardiovascular.

Vasovagal events are triggered (situational) events. They occur when emotional, heat, and orthostatic stress cause the parasympathetic nervous system to be overactive and lead to bradycardia and hypotension [81]. Vasovagal reactions can be induced by diverse stimuli, but when they occur after events such as infusions, injections, and skin prick testing, after exercise, or after a sting, the clinician must distinguish between a vasovagal reaction and an allergy to the foreign substance. Typically, vasovagal responses can be distinguished from anaphylaxis by multiple features (Table 7.3), especially bradycardia in vasovagal reactions and tachycardia in anaphylaxis. However, anaphylactic events can manifest with bradycardia [82, 83]. In general, vasovagal reactions are benign and can be managed with lifestyle modifications such as good hydration, movement of leg muscles to prevent venous

Table 7.3 Key features to distinguish vasovagal reactions from anaphylaxis

Feature	Vasovagal	Anaphylaxis
Usual precipitant	Emotional or orthostatic stress	Exposure to foreign substance (can be idiopathic)
Prodrome	Dizziness, light-headedness	Sense of impending doom
Timing	Immediate or even prior to procedure	Typically 5 minutes to 1 hour, may be biphasic
Skin	Pallor, diaphoresis	Erythema, pruritus, urticaria, and angioedema (note approximately 10% of anaphylaxis does not have skin symptoms)
Gastrointestinal	Nausea	Abdominal pain/cramping, vomiting, diarrhea
Respiratory	None	Sneezing, rhinitis, obstructive symptoms of wheeze, dyspnea
Cardiovascular	Bradycardia, hypotension	Typically tachycardia with hypotension although exceptions occur

pooling of the blood, and supine position during emotional stresses, but some patients with severe or refractory vasovagal reactions are candidates for medications or pacing [81].

A rare form of reflex syncope can be induced by swallowing which would link the episode to eating [84, 85]. To add to complexity, there are reports of swallow-induced syncope being associated with only specific foods such as acidic citrus fruits [86], and this phenomenon would need to be distinguished from a food allergy. Another type of situational syncope, post-exercise syncope, may be confused with exercise-induced anaphylaxis.

Seizures

Seizures have been reported in 1–2% of anaphylaxis [3] and may occur due to the hypoperfusion [87]. The recognition of anaphylaxis as the preceding event can guide the management of the patient.

An allergist evaluating a patient for transient loss of consciousness/syncope/seizures will need to also consider safety aspects such as whether the patient is fit to operate motorized equipment such as driving, as per their local regulations.

Shock

Anaphylaxis is a type of distributive shock, characterized by vasodilation which leads to hypotension and then, if severe anaphylaxis, organ damage. Sepsis is the most common cause of distributive shock [88] and has a wide differential diagnosis [89]. Rarer causes of distributive shock are spinal cord injury and capillary leak syndrome.

Other types of shock which may less commonly mimic anaphylaxis are cardiogenic, hypovolemic, and obstructive (e.g., pulmonary embolism, tension pneumothorax, cardiac tamponade) [3].

Cardiogenic shock derives special mention in the context of anaphylaxis. During anaphylaxis, cardiac mast cells can degranulate and lead to vasoconstriction and thrombosis. This hypersensitivity-associated myocardial involvement is called Kounis syndrome [90, 91]. In the type I variant of Kounis syndrome, allergic coronary artery spasm occurs with or without increase of cardiac enzymes and troponins. In the type II variant, coronary artery spasm occurs with plaque erosion or rupture manifesting as acute MI. The type III variant refers to patients with allergy-mediated coronary artery stent thrombosis [92]. Therefore, while cardiogenic shock can mimic anaphylaxis, cardiogenic shock can also be a consequence of anaphylaxis.

Shock has a wide differential diagnosis and requires resuscitation first and then considerations for the cause of the sepsis and ruling out mimickers [89].

Predominantly Gastrointestinal Symptoms

Gastrointestinal symptoms occur in 25–30% of anaphylaxis [3]. In addition to the conditions with flushing which can have prominent gastrointestinal symptoms such as NETs, there are some conditions with predominantly gastrointestinal symptoms which may be confused with anaphylaxis. Food poisoning will be considered under postprandial syndromes.

Abdominal Migraine/Cyclical Vomiting

Other syndromes which may be confused with anaphylaxis include abdominal migraine and cyclical vomiting [93].

Postprandial Syndromes

When significant symptoms occur in the setting of a meal, there may be more tendency to consider allergy and anaphylaxis as a cause. Therefore, it is helpful to consider specifically the postprandial masqueraders of anaphylaxis. As mentioned above, reflex syncope from swallowing and acute foreign body aspiration can mimic anaphylaxis.

Food Protein-Induced Enterocolitis Syndrome (FPIES)

Food protein-induced enterocolitis syndrome (FPIES) [94] is a non-IgE-mediated food allergy in which the hallmark is repeated vomiting beginning 1–4 hours after eating and symptoms often include lethargy, pallor, and diarrhea. The delay in onset and lack of urticaria or angioedema are helpful when distinguishing FPIES from anaphylaxis. However, these patients can have significant hypotension and be diagnosed as having shock. Laboratory tests can show methemoglobinemia and acidemia. FPIES is most common in infants but can be seen in adults. Furthermore, a milder chronic form can present with predominantly gastrointestinal symptoms. A subset of patients can have positive IgE tests to the culprit food or other foods which can further confuse the distinction between FPIES and anaphylaxis.

Food Poisoning

The food poisoning syndrome of scombroidosis is discussed in flushing. There are other foods which can give toxic effects and mimic anaphylaxis. One example is the Jamaican ackee fruit ("ishin" in Nigeria) which can give diarrhea and confusion secondary to hypoglycemia [95]. Mushroom toxicity can cause vomiting and diarrhea and lead to liver failure [96]. A detailed history of ingestions is central to the evaluation of suspected anaphylaxis.

Pollen-Food Allergy Syndrome

Pollen-food allergy syndrome is a food allergy occurring in pollen-allergic individuals. In pollen-food syndrome, there are predominantly local mouth symptoms upon eating fruits, vegetables, and nuts which have similarity to pollens [97]. Anaphylaxis can rarely occur.

Postprandial Hypoglycemia

Postprandial hypoglycemia can sometimes be mistaken for an allergic reaction to a food or medication. Symptoms which may mimic anaphylaxis include the classic hypoglycemia symptoms of tachycardia, anxiety, tremors, sweating, nausea, weakness, confusion, and light-headedness [98]. The demonstration of postprandial hypoglycemia requires fulfillment of Whipple's triad of (1) symptoms and/or signs of hypoglycemia, (2) documentation of low plasma glucose at the time of suspected hypoglycemia, and (3) correction of hypoglycemia resolves the symptoms/signs of hypoglycemia. If Whipple's triad is fulfilled, then a search for the cause of hypoglycemia is required and may include medications or a NET [98].

Non-organic Conditions

Non-organic conditions are also on the differential diagnosis of anaphylaxis. These conditions may be classified into involuntary and voluntary conditions. Involuntary anaphylaxis mimickers include panic attacks, somatization, and vocal cord dysfunction [3]. Munchausen stridor [1, 99, 100], now referred to as factitious disorder

[101], is a voluntary condition in which the patient is intentionally producing stridorous breathing by adducting their vocal cords. The stridor cannot be continued during coughing [3] which may help to distinguish this disorder from organic causes.

Summary

There are multiple conditions which can masquerade as anaphylaxis. A careful history of preceding events with particular attention to ingestions and stings, as well as details about symptoms present and pertinent negatives, can help to elucidate the cause of the event and differentiate the masqueraders of anaphylaxis from anaphylaxis.

References

1. Lieberman P, et al. Anaphylaxis – a practice parameter update 2015. Ann Allergy Asthma Immunol. 2015;115(5):341–84.
2. Tanno LK, et al. Critical view of anaphylaxis epidemiology: open questions and new perspectives. Allergy Asthma Clin Immunol. 2018;14:12.
3. Brown SGA, Kemp SF, Lieberman PL. 77 - Anaphylaxis. In: Adkinson NF, et al., editors. Middleton's allergy (Eighth Edition). London: 2014. p. 1237–59.
4. Sachar S, et al. Uncommon locations and presentations of hydatid cyst. Ann Med Health Sci Res. 2014;4(3):447–52.
5. Shimamura Y, et al. Common symptoms from an uncommon infection: gastrointestinal anisakiasis. Can J Gastroenterol Hepatol. 2016;2016:5176502.
6. Nieuwenhuizen NE, Lopata AL. Anisakis – a food-borne parasite that triggers allergic host defences. Int J Parasitol. 2013;43(12–13):1047–57.
7. Simons FE. Anaphylaxis. J Allergy Clin Immunol. 2010;125(2 Suppl 2):S161–81.
8. Koike T, et al. Brief report: severe symptoms of hyperhistaminemia after the treatment of acute promyelocytic leukemia with tretinoin (all-trans-retinoic acid). N Engl J Med. 1992;327(6):385–7.
9. Ching JC, et al. Peanut and fish allergy due to platelet transfusion in a child. CMAJ. 2015;187(12):905–7.
10. Arnold DM, et al. Passive transfer of peanut hypersensitivity by fresh frozen plasma. Arch Intern Med. 2007;167(8):853–4.
11. Valent P, et al. Advances in the classification and treatment of mastocytosis: current status and outlook toward the future. Cancer Res. 2017;77(6):1261–70.
12. Bonadonna P, Scaffidi L. Hymenoptera anaphylaxis as a clonal mast cell disorder. Immunol Allergy Clin N Am. 2018;38(3):455–68.
13. Gulen T, et al. The presence of mast cell clonality in patients with unexplained anaphylaxis. Clin Exp Allergy. 2014;44(9):1179–87.
14. Gulen T, et al. High prevalence of anaphylaxis in patients with systemic mastocytosis - a single-centre experience. Clin Exp Allergy. 2014;44(1):121–9.
15. Akin C. Anaphylaxis and mast cell disease: what is the risk? Curr Allergy Asthma Rep. 2010;10(1):34–8.
16. Pardanani A. Systemic mastocytosis in adults: 2019 update on diagnosis, risk stratification and management. Am J Hematol. 2019;94(3):363–77. https://doi.org/10.1002/ajh.25371.
17. Hamilton MJ. Nonclonal mast cell activation syndrome: a growing body of evidence. Immunol Allergy Clin N Am. 2018;38(3):469–81.

18. Akin C. Mast cell activation syndromes presenting as anaphylaxis. Immunol Allergy Clin N Am. 2015;35(2):277–85.
19. Zuberbier T, et al. The EAACI/GA(2)LEN/EDF/WAO guideline for the definition, classification, diagnosis and management of urticaria. Allergy. 2018;73(7):1393–414.
20. Davis MDP, van der Hilst JCH. Mimickers of urticaria: urticarial vasculitis and autoinflammatory diseases. J Allergy Clin Immunol Pract. 2018;6(4):1162–70.
21. Dreyfus DH. Differential diagnosis of chronic urticaria and angioedema based on molecular biology, pharmacology, and proteomics. Immunol Allergy Clin N Am. 2017;37(1):201–15.
22. Maurer M, Fluhr JW, Khan DA. How to approach chronic inducible urticaria. J Allergy Clin Immunol Pract. 2018;6(4):1119–30.
23. Jung WS, Kim SH, Lee H. Missed diagnosis of anaphylaxis in patients with pediatric urticaria in emergency department. Pediatr Emerg Care. 2018 Oct 2. https://doi.org/10.1097/PEC.0000000000001617.
24. Gill P, Betschel SD. The clinical evaluation of angioedema. Immunol Allergy Clin N Am. 2017;37(3):449–66.
25. Kaplan AP, Joseph K. Pathogenesis of hereditary angioedema: the role of the bradykinin-forming cascade. Immunol Allergy Clin N Am. 2017;37(3):513–25.
26. Farkas H, et al. International consensus on the diagnosis and management of pediatric patients with hereditary angioedema with C1 inhibitor deficiency. Allergy. 2017;72(2):300–13.
27. Otani IM, Banerji A. Acquired C1 inhibitor deficiency. Immunol Allergy Clin N Am. 2017;37(3):497–511.
28. Bas M. The angiotensin-converting-enzyme-induced angioedema. Immunol Allergy Clin N Am. 2017;37(1):183–200.
29. Stone C Jr, Brown NJ. Angiotensin-converting enzyme inhibitor and other drug-associated angioedema. Immunol Allergy Clin N Am. 2017;37(3):483–95.
30. Kowalski ML, Woessner K, Sanak M. Approaches to the diagnosis and management of patients with a history of nonsteroidal anti-inflammatory drug-related urticaria and angioedema. J Allergy Clin Immunol. 2015;136(2):245–51.
31. Huston DP, Sabato V. Decoding the enigma of urticaria and angioedema. J Allergy Clin Immunol Pract. 2018;6(4):1171–5.
32. Magerl M, et al. Hereditary angioedema with normal C1 inhibitor: update on evaluation and treatment. Immunol Allergy Clin N Am. 2017;37(3):571–84.
33. Weston WL. EPP masquerading as angioedema. J Allergy Clin Immunol. 1978;61(6):408.
34. Bova M, et al. Hereditary and acquired angioedema: heterogeneity of pathogenesis and clinical phenotypes. Int Arch Allergy Immunol. 2018;175(3):126–35.
35. Wu MA, et al. Angioedema phenotypes: disease expression and classification. Clin Rev Allergy Immunol. 2016;51(2):162–9.
36. Farkas H, et al. "Nuts and bolts" of laboratory evaluation of angioedema. Clin Rev Allergy Immunol. 2016;51(2):140–51.
37. Hannah-Shmouni F, Stratakis CA, Koch CA. Flushing in (neuro)endocrinology. Rev Endocr Metab Disord. 2016;17(3):373–80.
38. Huguet I, Grossman A. Management of Endocrine Disease: Flushing: current concepts. Eur J Endocrinol. 2017;177(5):R219–29.
39. Sadeghian A, et al. Etiologies and management of cutaneous flushing: malignant causes. J Am Acad Dermatol. 2017;77(3):405–14.
40. Rastogi V, et al. Flushing disorders associated with gastrointestinal symptoms: part 2, systemic miscellaneous conditions. Clin Med Res. 2018;16(1–2):29–36.
41. Rastogi V, et al. Flushing disorders associated with gastrointestinal symptoms: part 1, neuroendocrine tumors, mast cell disorders and hyperbasophila. Clin Med Res. 2018;16(1–2):16–28.
42. Izikson L, English JC 3rd, Zirwas MJ. The flushing patient: differential diagnosis, workup, and treatment. J Am Acad Dermatol. 2006;55(2):193–208.
43. Davison AS, et al. Clinical evaluation and treatment of phaeochromocytoma. Ann Clin Biochem. 2018;55(1):34–48.

44. Lenders JW, et al. Pheochromocytoma and paraganglioma: an endocrine society clinical practice guideline. J Clin Endocrinol Metab. 2014;99(6):1915–42.
45. Sadeghian A, et al. Etiologies and management of cutaneous flushing: nonmalignant causes. J Am Acad Dermatol. 2017;77(3):391–402.
46. Fertleman CR, et al. Paroxysmal extreme pain disorder (previously familial rectal pain syndrome). Neurology. 2007;69(6):586–95.
47. Avgerinos DV, Theoharides TC. Mesenteric traction syndrome or gut in distress. Int J Immunopathol Pharmacol. 2005;18(2):195–9.
48. Bradberry SM, et al. Poisoning due to pyrethroids. Toxicol Rev. 2005;24(2):93–106.
49. Oronsky B, et al. Nothing but NET: a review of neuroendocrine tumors and carcinomas. Neoplasia. 2017;19(12):991–1002.
50. Fagin JA, Wells SA Jr. Biologic and clinical perspectives on thyroid cancer. N Engl J Med. 2016;375(23):2307.
51. Raue F, Frank-Raue K. Update on multiple endocrine neoplasia type 2: focus on medullary thyroid carcinoma. J Endocrinol Soc. 2018;2(8):933–43.
52. Vogel WH. Infusion reactions: diagnosis, assessment, and management. Clin J Oncol Nurs. 2010;14(2):E10–21.
53. Burke MJ, Rheingold SR. Differentiating hypersensitivity versus infusion-related reactions in pediatric patients receiving intravenous asparaginase therapy for acute lymphoblastic leukemia. Leuk Lymphoma. 2017;58(3):540–51.
54. Ridolo E, et al. Scombroid syndrome: it seems to be fish allergy but... it isn't. Curr Opin Allergy Clin Immunol. 2016;16(5):516–21.
55. Anagnostou K, Turner PJ. Myths, facts and controversies in the diagnosis and management of anaphylaxis. Arch Dis Child. 2019;104(1):83–90.
56. Kann K, Long B, Koyfman A. Clinical mimics: an emergency medicine-focused review of asthma mimics. J Emerg Med. 2017;53(2):195–201.
57. Foong RX, du Toit G, Fox AT. Mini review - asthma and food allergy. Curr Pediatr Rev. 2018;14(3):164–70.
58. Caffarelli C, et al. Asthma and food allergy in children: is there a connection or interaction? Front Pediatr. 2016;4:34.
59. Akenroye AT, et al. Prevalence of anaphylaxis among adults admitted to critical care for severe asthma exacerbation. Emerg Med J. 2018;35(10):623–5.
60. Simons FE, et al. World allergy organization guidelines for the assessment and management of anaphylaxis. World Allergy Organ J. 2011;4(2):13–37.
61. Muglia C, Oppenheimer J. Wheezing in infancy: an overview of recent literature. Curr Allergy Asthma Rep. 2017;17(10):67.
62. Fretzayas A, et al. Differentiating vocal cord dysfunction from asthma. J Asthma Allergy. 2017;10:277–83.
63. Nugent JS, et al. Levothyroxine anaphylaxis? Vocal cord dysfunction mimicking an anaphylactic drug reaction. Ann Allergy Asthma Immunol. 2003;91(4):337–41.
64. Garcia-Neuer M, et al. Drug-induced paradoxical vocal fold motion. J Allergy Clin Immunol Pract. 2018;6(1):90–4.
65. Ahrens B, et al. Think twice: misleading food-induced respiratory symptoms in children with food allergy. Pediatr Pulmonol. 2014;49(3):E59–62.
66. Kjaer HF, et al. Venom anaphylaxis can mimic other serious conditions and disclose important underlying disease. Ann Allergy Asthma Immunol. 2018;120(3):338–9.
67. Gee MR, Kruyer WB. Case report of an aviator with a single episode of altered consciousness due to Hymenoptera hypersensitivity. Aviat Space Environ Med. 1999;70(11):1113–6.
68. Robles LA, Matilla AF. Brain stem ischemic stroke associated with anaphylaxis. Cureus. 2018;10(3):e2289.
69. Johnson JA, et al. Thromboembolic stroke: a sequela of Hymenoptera venom-induced anaphylaxis. Ann Allergy Asthma Immunol. 2016;116(3):262–4.
70. Kulhari A, et al. Ischemic stroke after wasp sting. J Emerg Med. 2016;51(4):405–10.

71. Brignole M. *'Ten Commandments' of ESC Syncope Guidelines* 2018: The new European Society of Cardiology (ESC) Clinical Practice Guidelines for the diagnosis and management of syncope were launched 19 March 2018 at EHRA 2018 in Barcelona. Eur Heart J. 2018;39(21):1870–1.
72. Corrigendum to: 2018 ESC Guidelines for the diagnosis and management of syncope. Eur Heart J. 2018;39(21):2002.
73. Brignole M, et al. 2018 ESC Guidelines for the diagnosis and management of syncope. Eur Heart J. 2018;39(21):1883–948.
74. Brignole M, et al. Practical Instructions for the 2018 ESC Guidelines for the diagnosis and management of syncope. Eur Heart J. 2018;39(21):e43–80.
75. Reed MJ. Approach to syncope in the emergency department. Emerg Med J. 2019;36(2):108–16.
76. Schunk PC, Ruttan T. Pediatric syncope: high-risk conditions and reasonable approach. Emerg Med Clin North Am. 2018;36(2):305–21.
77. Coleman DK, Long B, Koyfman A. Clinical mimics: an emergency medicine-focused review of syncope mimics. J Emerg Med. 2018;54(1):81–9.
78. Fant C, Cohen A, Vazquez MN. Syncope in pediatric patients: a practical approach to differential diagnosis and management in the emergency department [digest]. Pediatr Emerg Med Pract. 2017;14(4 Suppl Points & Pearls):S1–2.
79. Fant C, Cohen A. Syncope in pediatric patients: a practical approach to differential diagnosis and management in the emergency department. Pediatr Emerg Med Pract. 2017;14(4):1–28.
80. Runser LA, Gauer RL, Houser A. Syncope: evaluation and differential diagnosis. Am Fam Physician. 2017;95(5):303–12.
81. Kenny RA, McNicholas T. The management of vasovagal syncope. QJM. 2016;109(12):767–73.
82. Simon MR. Anaphylaxis associated with relative bradycardia. Ann Allergy. 1989;62(6):495–7.
83. Brown SG. Anaphylaxis: clinical concepts and research priorities. Emerg Med Australas. 2006;18(2):155–69.
84. Kohno R, et al. Swallow (deglutition) syncope: an evaluation of swallowing-induced heart rate and hemodynamic changes in affected patients and control subjects. J Cardiovasc Electrophysiol. 2019;30(2):221–9.
85. Aydogdu I, et al. Swallow-induced syncope in 5 patients: electrophysiologic evaluation during swallowing. Neurol Clin Pract. 2017;7(4):316–23.
86. Yamaguchi Y, et al. Citrus fruits induced swallow syncope with atrioventricular block or sinus arrest. J Electrocardiol. 2018;51(4):613–6.
87. Kharal GA, Darby RR, Cohen AB. Envenomation seizures. Neurohospitalist. 2018;8(1):29–30.
88. Alyesil C, et al. Distributive shock in the emergency department: sepsis, anaphylaxis, or capillary leak syndrome? J Emerg Med. 2017;52(6):e229–31.
89. Long B, Koyfman A. Clinical mimics: an emergency medicine-focused review of sepsis mimics. J Emerg Med. 2017;52(1):34–42.
90. Kounis NG, et al. Anaphylactic cardiovascular collapse and Kounis syndrome: systemic vasodilation or coronary vasoconstriction? Ann Transl Med. 2018;6(17):332.
91. Abdelghany M, et al. Kounis syndrome: a review article on epidemiology, diagnostic findings, management and complications of allergic acute coronary syndrome. Int J Cardiol. 2017;232:1–4.
92. Kounis NG. Kounis syndrome: an update on epidemiology, pathogenesis, diagnosis and therapeutic management. Clin Chem Lab Med. 2016;54(10):1545–59.
93. Irwin S, Barmherzig R, Gelfand A. Recurrent gastrointestinal disturbance: abdominal migraine and cyclic vomiting syndrome. Curr Neurol Neurosci Rep. 2017;17(3):21.
94. Nowak-Wegrzyn A, et al. International consensus guidelines for the diagnosis and management of food protein-induced enterocolitis syndrome: Executive summary-Workgroup Report of the Adverse Reactions to Foods Committee, American Academy of Allergy, Asthma & Immunology. J Allergy Clin Immunol. 2017;139(4):1111–26. e4
95. Katibi OS, et al. Ackee fruit poisoning in eight siblings: implications for public health awareness. Am J Trop Med Hyg. 2015;93(5):1122–3.

96. Vanooteghem S, et al. Four patients with Amanita Phalloides poisoning. Acta Gastroenterol Belg. 2014;77(3):353–6.
97. Webber CM, England RW. Oral allergy syndrome: a clinical, diagnostic, and therapeutic challenge. Ann Allergy Asthma Immunol. 2010;104(2):101–8; quiz 109–10, 117.
98. Kittah NE, Vella A. Management of Endocrine Disease: pathogenesis and management of hypoglycemia. Eur J Endocrinol. 2017;177(1):R37–47.
99. Bahna SL, Oldham JL. Munchausen stridor-a strong false alarm of anaphylaxis. Allergy Asthma Immunol Res. 2014;6(6):577–9.
100. Wong HC. Factitious anaphylaxis and pre-varication anaphylaxis. J Allergy Clin Immunol. 2005;116(3):710. author reply 710
101. Jafferany M, et al. Psychological aspects of factitious disorder. Prim Care Companion CNS Disord. 2018;20(1).

Anaphylaxis Education: For Patients, Daycares, Schools, and Colleges

Nicole B. Ramsey and Julie Wang

Introduction

Anaphylaxis is a life-threatening systemic allergic reaction that affects 0.05–2% of the population in the United States [1] and 3% of the population in Europe [2]. Most times, a trigger is not identified [3]; however, when a trigger is known, it may include food, insect sting, medication, or exercise. Food is the most common trigger in school-aged children [4].

Food allergy in children is reported in approximately 8% of children in the United States, and 40% of these children have been cited as having a severe reaction (including anaphylaxis) [5]. Not only is food allergy relatively common, its prevalence has also been noted to increase over time, 18% in 10 years in the United States (1997–2007) [6].

Reactions Often Occur at School

Children spend most of their time at school, and the frequency of reactions at school has been studied both in the United and States and abroad. Of children who have anaphylaxis events, 25–50% of initial reactions (treated by an epinephrine auto-injector, EAI) occur while at school [7, 8]. Sixteen to eighteen percent of schools surveyed by the EpiPen4Schools® program, an initiative to help provide unassigned EAIs to schools in the United States, reported episodes of anaphylaxis from 2013 to 2015 [9, 10]. Within the school day in the United States, reactions can occur in the classroom (65–83%), lunchroom (10–19%), field trips/commute (5–19%), playground (10–19%), or gymnasium (9%) [7, 9, 11–14]. In Western Australia, 1 in 7

N. B. Ramsey · J. Wang (✉)
Department of Pediatrics, Division of Allergy and Immunology, Icahn School of Medicine at Mount Sinai, New York, NY, USA
e-mail: Nicole.ramsey@mountsinai.org; Julie.wang@mssm.edu

© Springer Nature Switzerland AG 2020
A. K. Ellis (ed.), *Anaphylaxis*, https://doi.org/10.1007/978-3-030-43205-8_8

schools and 1 in 30 daycares reported having anaphylaxis occurring to a student on-site in 2008 [15]. In the European Anaphylaxis Registry from 2007 to 2015, anaphylaxis cases occurred about 9% of the time at school [16].

Data on this subject, although valuable, is limited by the type of study, which ranges from cross-sectional paper or telephone surveys that rely on recollection of parents to EAI reporting database analysis, which only includes those reactions treated with an EAI as a surrogate measure of anaphylaxis.

Risk Factors

In general, anaphylaxis carries most risk in infants, teenagers, pregnant women, and the elderly [17]. Comorbidities like asthma, mast cell disorders (particularly for venom allergy), and cardiovascular disease also pose an increased risk for more severe allergic symptoms [18–20]. Medications (NSAIDs, alcohol use) and other host factors (exercise, stress, menstruation) may also lower allergic thresholds [21].

These risk factors uniquely affect adolescents/college students, toddlers/preschool children, and children with multiple food allergies. Adolescent risks include decreased vigilance about avoiding their allergen trigger, increased risk-taking behaviors, decreased likelihood of carrying their EAIs, worry about embarrassment about reactions around their peers, and impaired judgment due to experimenting with drugs and alcohol [22]. They also distinctively encounter the decreased threshold associated with exercise, stress, and menstruation as these may occur at high frequency or levels and may occur for the first time in adolescence. As shown by McWilliam et al. in 2018, adolescents, particularly with multiple allergies, tend to have more frequent reactions [22]. Young children under 5 years have the most frequent, albeit less severe, reactions compared to children of other ages [22]. They are less verbal and therefore more likely to have accidental exposure because of messy eating and mouthing toys [23–25].

Triggers

Anaphylaxis triggers are not always identified. When triggers are identified, they are most commonly foods in children, while medication or insect venom allergy more often occurs in adults [4]. Of course, any trigger can affect any individual, regardless of age. Food-induced anaphylaxis affects children at school and can be triggered in many instances by peanuts (all ages), milk or egg (young children), and shellfish (older children) [5]. Other common triggers include wheat, soy, tree nuts, and finned fish. Medication triggers include antibiotics, NSAIDs, contrast agents, biologic agents, chemotherapies, vaccines, and allergen immunotherapy [4, 26]. Medication-induced anaphylaxis is less likely to occur at school, unless children are taking scheduled medications during the school day or attend school-based health clinics. Insect sting anaphylaxis can occur and contributes to up to 0.8% of anaphylaxis cases in children [4, 27]. One study in the United States documented that 1/3 of cases occurred at school and 2/3 occurred while out with family and friends [28].

Venom anaphylaxis, although rare in children, can occur on school grounds, such as on the playground or sports fields.

Reducing the Risk of Allergen Exposure

The most important measure for anaphylaxis prevention is allergen avoidance. For food allergy, avoidance includes label reading for all food products and taking care when preparing food to avoid cross-contamination. Of note, the main risk with food allergy is by the oral route of exposure, while skin and inhalation risks are less likely to cause severe reactions for most allergens. Healthcare professionals, schools, and families should work collaboratively to help students be prepared for reactions which may occur during school or at school-related events [7] since accidental exposures can occur despite allergen avoidance efforts. In particular, healthcare professionals should provide families with accurate diagnoses and evidence-based recommendations for management, assist families and schools in developing management plans, and encourage families to provide up-to-date information and emergency medications to schools.

Training of Staff at School

School staff must be appropriately trained to recognize allergic reactions, administer EAIs, and be knowledgeable about existing school policies [15, 29]. Annual training for school staff, including nurses and teachers, can be beneficial [30], and more frequent training may be needed for daycare centers which often have high staff turnover [31].One reason that staff members besides nurses should be trained is a lack of nurse availability and proximity to allergic reactions in many schools. In fact, teachers administer the EAI in 59% of cases according to a study by Sicherer et al. [12]. Having more staff available to respond quickly to allergic reactions can prevent delays in EAI administration, which has been linked to poorer outcomes [32].

There is significant variability of who is trained to treat anaphylaxis at schools [10]. Training improves attitude and knowledge about allergic reactions as shown in several studies around the world [33–36]. A number of resources have been developed to support training for staff and students at daycare, school, or college [37–40].

Safety Measures in Classrooms, Lunchrooms, and Sports Fields

Classrooms are the location where food-allergic reactions occur most frequently in school [12]. In this setting, reactions can occur due to crafts (examples include wheat in finger paint and Play-Doh, milk in shaving cream and finger paint, nuts and/or seeds in bird feed) and celebrations with food. When cleaning surfaces contaminated with crafts and/or foods, soap and water or wipes are the methods of choice; they are superior to hand sanitizer in removing allergenic proteins [41].

Still, the most common source of food-induced anaphylaxis is by oral ingestion of foods and not by cutaneous exposure or inhalation [42, 43].

Some schools have chosen to implement policies restricting allergenic foods; approaches include no sharing policies, nonfood classroom activities or celebrations, and wider restrictions, either from the entire school or from specific areas of the school. Another strategy schools have implemented to prevent food-allergic reactions is to have designated areas in the lunchroom that are allergen restricted. In one study, this has been linked to decreased EAI use [44]. However, concerns about this approach include isolation of allergic students and feasibility when multiple food allergies or allergies to staple foods like milk and egg are involved. Overall, there is limited data to support the effectiveness of these approaches in reducing accidental allergen exposures or rates of allergic reactions [45–47].

Anaphylaxis can occur outside the classroom and lunchroom as well, including on the sports fields, during field trips, and on school buses. This is of particular concern for insect sting anaphylaxis. The Australasian Society of Clinical Immunology and Allergy (ASCIA) guidelines recommend that schools: identify low-risk play areas (away from plants and gardens known to attract stinging insects), ensure students are properly covered while outside (to prevent fire ant bites), and avoid open containers (that might attract wasps) [15]. Trained staff and emergency medication should also be readily available in these areas.

Special Populations and Considerations

There are special considerations regarding young children and adolescents with anaphylaxis. Anaphylaxis occurs most frequently in children who are preschool age, and this rate is increasing more quickly than in other age groups [48]. Toddlers are not able to comprehend or comply with the rules about food sharing, may have limited ability to verbalize allergy symptoms, more commonly participate in crafts that may contain food ingredients, and have mouthing behaviors that can pose a risk for allergen exposure (such as mouthing toys and surfaces, thumb sucking) [49]. Preschools and daycare centers should label cups and bottles to prevent sharing and clean toys and surfaces to remove contamination [31].

Adolescents also deserve increased attention as they tend to have more severe allergic reactions [5]. Adolescents are more prone to risk-taking due to peer pressure and newfound independence. They treat anaphylaxis with EAIs less commonly than other age groups and are less likely to self-carry EAIs due to inconvenience or embarrassment [50, 51]. Young adults are often experimenting with alcohol and drugs (lowers allergy thresholds and impairs judgment) and intimacy (kissing could expose them to allergens through saliva). Allergists and pediatricians should educate young adults regarding these types of management concerns as they may be unaware of the risks. In addition to less preparation and increased likelihood of allergen exposure, adolescents often underestimate the severity of their symptoms [51].

Whether it's an adolescent choosing a college or a mom choosing a daycare, there are special considerations for allergic children and families. Table 8.1 describes

Table 8.1 Reducing risk and optimizing care for students at risk for anaphylaxis in daycares, schools, and college

Allergen avoidance	• Food allergy
	  – Consider allergen-free art/science projects and celebrations
	  – Consider policies to limit sharing of foods and cups/bottles (in daycares)
	  – Routine cleaning of surfaces and toys
	  – Label reading for packaged foods served by the school and education on cross-contact for food services staff
	• Insect sting allergy
	  – Identify low-risk outdoor play areas
	  – Remove any nests in areas near school

Managing allergic reactions	• Emergency medications (epinephrine auto-injectors) should be readily available and accessible
	• Families should provide updated medical information provided to appropriate school staff (emergency action plan)
	• Ensure availability of trained staff who can recognize signs and symptoms of allergic reactions
	• Staff should be knowledgeable about school policies related to anaphylaxis
	• Preparation and adequate staffing during off-site activities (i.e., field trips, sporting events)
	• Encourage self-carrying of epinephrine auto-injectors, if developmentally appropriate
	• Adolescents should be guided closely due to
	  – Lower thresholds due to drugs or alcohol
	  – More severe reactions due to risk-taking and peer pressure
	  – Less willingness to carry EAIs due to inconvenience and embarrassment

key points for healthcare providers to discuss allergen avoidance and reaction management with families needing to make these decisions [52].

One qualitative study at college campuses found that notifying others in the student's campus network about food allergy, establishing clearly defined roles/responsibilities, and broadening campus awareness of food allergy and the potential consequences of accidental exposure are the most important for improving food allergy management [53]. Another epidemiologic survey showed improvements at one university after implementation of a program for comprehensive food allergy dietary/nutritional support and dining hall labeling [54]. Improvements were seen in contacts being aware of food allergy (20% improvement), dining hall labeling for allergen content (150% improvement), avoiding food allergen (25% improvement), EAI carrying (409% improvement), and maintaining EAI (75% improvement) [54].

Preparedness and Management of Allergic Reactions

Timely administration of epinephrine for anaphylaxis improves outcomes. Therefore, having ready access to epinephrine is important. Individuals with known allergy who are prescribed EAIs should provide them to the schools or self-carry, if developmentally appropriate. Where available, stock epinephrine is also important for treating those with first-time allergic reactions and those with known allergy who do not have EAIs available (or who require multiple epinephrine injections) [55].

To guide staff, teachers, and school nurses, emergency action plans and medication administration forms specifying known triggers, dose, and symptoms should be submitted by families annually to school nursing. Notably, in a study in NYC (2007–2013), allergic children who identify as Black or Asian are two to three times less likely to have a medication administration form submitted before requiring EAI administration at school [56]. In this same study, after unknown trigger, food was the next most common.

Treatment Barriers

Barriers to treatment include lack of access to EAI because there is no stock available, a student with known allergy doesn't self-carry or hasn't provided an EAI to the school, the EAI is inaccessible or the EAI is not administered due to fear or uncertainty, as well as hesitancy to call emergency services in the face of a reaction [31, 56, 57].

Schools should ensure that EAIs are kept in an easily accessible locations [58]. In most (56%) US schools, persons other than nurses are only allowed to give an EAI when the person reacting has a known allergic diagnosis [59]. However, only about half of schools in one study of over 12,000 schools had full-time school nurses [9].

School Plans and Protections

Individualized health plans (IHPs) include an emergency action plan for a student, education for the school, and appropriate avoidance measures for the student. It should also address sports and field trips, medication access, cafeterias, and transportation.

Section 504 of the US rehabilitation Act of 1973 bans discrimination against persons with disabilities in any activity or program which receives federal funding [60]. According to this legislation, 504 plans can be created for detailed documentation of agreements regarding accommodation that cannot be covered in an IHP. 504 plans may be especially important for children who need help with reading food labels or need developmentally appropriate guidance with avoiding allergens.

Psychosocial Factors

The psychosocial impact on children at risk for anaphylaxis has mostly been studied in patients with food allergy. Quality of life has been reported by survey to be worse for food allergy patients than those with other chronic illnesses like diabetes and cardiovascular disease [61–63]. This may be due to increased stress (9–41%) and/or social isolation (49%) [63, 64]. Bullying can also impact quality of life, and there is emerging data demonstrating that food-allergic children are experiencing bullying at higher rates than children who are not food allergic [65, 66]. Food allergy-related bullying occurs at school (86% of cases) and includes not only verbal acts (64%) but also physical harassment (57%). Teachers are cited as perpetrators in 21% of cases [65]. Bullying is not well-recognized – 53% of teachers acknowledge that children with food allergy are at risk for bullying and 4% of teachers reported being aware that food-allergic students experienced bullying in their own classroom [67].

These impacts are not always apparent [68], and bullying in general has been associated with decreased school performance [69]. Therefore, physicians should regularly ask about these during office visits. Physicians and parents should also consider mental health resources when bullying or anxiety related to food allergies requires professional support.

Roles and Responsibilities

Importance of Collaboration

Effective teamwork, timely communication, and collaboration among physicians, school staff, caregivers, and students are crucial for children at risk for anaphylaxis (Fig. 8.1) [70].

Caregiver

Caregivers are at the crux of communication and must learn about allergy management from physicians and ensure schools have necessary medications and up-to-date medical information [71].

Physician

The pediatrician and allergist can educate and prepare patients and their families to manage allergic reactions in the school setting. In addition, they can engage in advocacy work to collaborate with schools to support school staff training and develop policies for anaphylaxis management.

School Nurse

The school nurse should collaborate with physicians to provide individualized care according to healthcare plans. They are the main healthcare professionals on-site at schools, and they coordinate care, advocate for direct student needs, respond to emergencies, and educate staff, students, and families [30]. The nurse can also

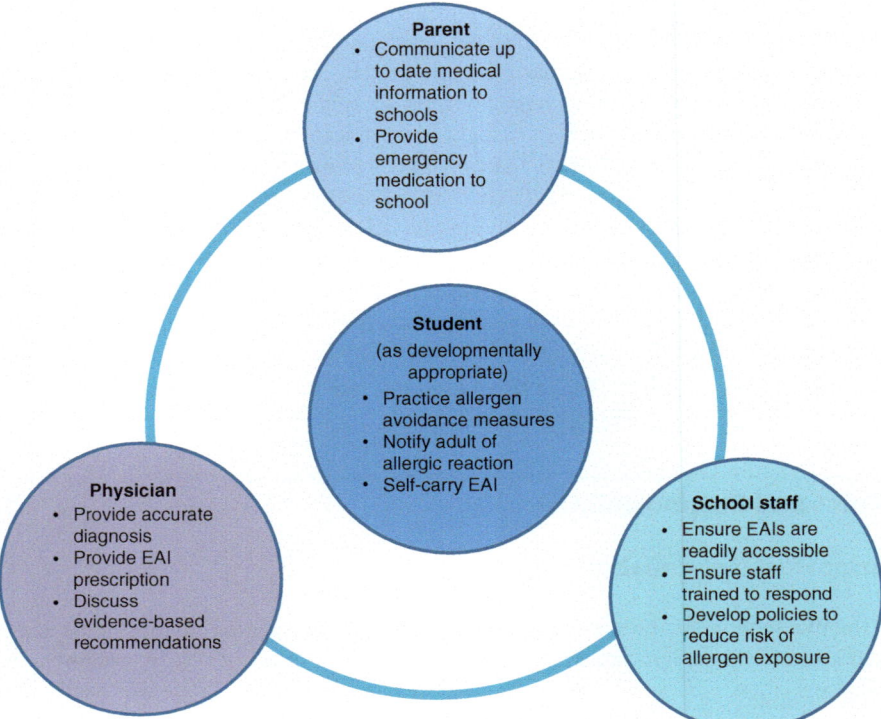

Fig. 8.1 Teamwork and communication between the student, caregiver, school staff, and the physician is at the crux of good care and emergency management for anaphylaxis at daycare, school, and college

ensure that emergency medicines are readily accessible within minutes to vulnerable students during the school day [58].

School Staff

Non-nursing school staff may be the first responder in an anaphylaxis emergency and should be trained to recognize the signs and symptoms of allergic reactions, administer an EAI, and/or call for help. They can help create safe learning environments for at-risk students by limiting or avoiding the use of known allergens in school-related activities.

Student

Over time as the student becomes more developmentally and cognitively mature, they should practice allergen avoidance measures, quickly inform school staff about any symptoms, self-carry EAIs, and be trained to self-administer medications in the event of an emergency.

Legislation and Guidelines

Legislation and Regulations

A number of global governments have enacted laws to support patients with life-threatening allergy by providing access to lifesaving EAIs at school or giving schools a guide for managing anaphylaxis/food allergy.

In 2011, the US Food Allergy and Anaphylaxis Management Act became law and mandated the development of voluntary school food allergy and anaphylaxis management guidelines by the US Secretary of Health and Human Services and the US Secretary of the Department of Education. Following this, the Centers for Disease Control and Prevention published the comprehensive voluntary guidelines for food allergy management in schools' document in 2013 to help guide schools with five priority areas: individual food allergy management, preparation for allergic emergencies (including anaphylaxis), food allergy training/professional development for staff, food allergy education for students and families, and healthy and safe educational environments [40]. The Americans with Disabilities Act of 1990 and its amendments (ADAA) in 2018 also protect children with food allergies and anaphylaxis who attend federally funded schools or nonreligious private schools [72]. The ADAA allows eligible students to have free dietary substitutions in school meal programs with written notice from a physician [60]. In November 2013, former President Barack Obama signed the School Access to Emergency Epinephrine Act, which encourages states to adopt laws requiring schools to keep stock epinephrine. In states where stock epinephrine is recommended by state law, there is varied uptake at schools (with decreased stock epinephrine in areas of lower socioeconomic status) [65], different rules for who is allowed to administer the EAI, and diverse guidance regarding reporting of allergic reactions and epinephrine use [58].

In Australia, Ministerial Order 706 mandates that public and private schools with enrolled students at risk for anaphylaxis develop a management policy; review emergency action plans (EAPs); train school staff routinely in the management; purchase stock EAIs; complete an annual anaphylaxis risk management checklist; develop a communication plan about anaphylaxis and school anaphylaxis policies for staff, students, and parents; identify prevention strategies to minimize anaphylaxis risk; and develop emergency protocols for anaphylaxis response. Stock epinephrine is mandated for use in all schools in Australia [66], and the country is also one of the first nations to have preschool/childcare-specific legislation for anaphylaxis. The National Quality Framework (2013) requires all schools to have trained educators in first aid and asthma and anaphylaxis management [66].

Recognition of the need to protect vulnerable children at risk for anaphylaxis is occurring in other countries as well. The Canadian School Boards Association has voluntary food allergy guidelines [67], and Ontario has a mandate known as

Sabrina's Law (An Act to Protect Anaphylactic Pupils 2006), which requires ana-phylaxis policy and individual healthcare plans for students at risk [66]. In 2015, the United Kingdom enacted a statutory guide under the Children and Families Act of 2014 which requires children to have an individualized healthcare plan if they have medical needs (including anaphylaxis) [66]. In 2011, The Ministry of Health, Labor and Welfare in Japan published the "Guideline on Measures Against Allergy at Nursery" and the "Certificate for Nursery Life Management." These guidelines along with the "Certificate for School Life Management" are being used to maintain a philosophy and methods of anaphylaxis management in the school setting [73].

Professional Guidelines

In addition to legislation, there are a number of guidelines for anaphylaxis manage-ment published by national/international medical organizations:

- The American Academy of Allergy, Asthma and Immunology published a posi-tion statement in 1998 entitled "Anaphylaxis in school and other childcare set-tings" to ameliorate the fatal risks of anaphylaxis described by Sampson et al. in 1992 [32, 74].
- The American Academy of Pediatrics published two guidelines in 2017 to guide physicians in creating an emergency action plan for patients at risk for anaphy-laxis and to guide them in prescribing EAIs when appropriate and educating families and patients about treatment of anaphylaxis with EAIs [75, 76].
- The Australasian Society of Clinical Immunology and Allergy has developed guidelines for the prevention of anaphylaxis in schools, preschools, and child-care (most recently updated in 2015), describing management principles for training, treatment, specific ages, initial reactions, and practical strategies [77].
- In 2014, the European Academy of Allergy and Clinical Immunology guidelines recommended that school principals be in charge of the implementation of a food allergy policy that ensures emergency action plan (EAP) development for affected children and training of teachers and staff to recognize allergies [78].

Conclusions

Anaphylaxis, a life-threatening systemic allergic reaction, can occur at school and may occur with increased frequency in toddlers and severity in adolescents. Schools should take measures to minimize risk of allergic reactions, and school staff should be trained to identify signs and symptoms of allergic reactions and to promptly administer epinephrine auto-injector(s) in case of severe reactions. Collaboration between students, families, school staff, and physicians facilitates effective care of those at risk for anaphylaxis. A number of resources and legislative measures exist to support families, daycares/schools/colleges, and physicians in the management of anaphylaxis to reduce risk and optimize outcomes.

References

1. Lieberman P, et al. Epidemiology of anaphylaxis: findings of the American College of Allergy, Asthma and Immunology Epidemiology of Anaphylaxis Working Group. Ann Allergy Asthma Immunol. 2006;97(5):596–602.
2. Panesar SS, et al. The epidemiology of anaphylaxis in Europe: a systematic review. Allergy. 2013;68(11):1353–61.
3. Lieberman PL. Idiopathic anaphylaxis. Allergy Asthma Proc. 2014;35(1):17–23.
4. Wood RA, et al. Anaphylaxis in America: the prevalence and characteristics of anaphylaxis in the United States. J Allergy Clin Immunol. 2014;133(2):461–7.
5. Gupta RS, et al. The prevalence, severity, and distribution of childhood food allergy in the United States. Pediatrics. 2011;128(1):e9–17.
6. Branum AM, Lukacs SL. Food allergy among children in the United States. Pediatrics. 2009;124(6):1549–55.
7. McIntyre CL, Sheetz AH, Carroll CR, Young MC. Administration of epinephrine for life-threatening allergic reactions in school settings. Pediatrics. 2005;116(5):1134–40.
8. Pouessel G, Lejeune S, Dupond M-P, Renard A, Fallot C, Deschildre A. Individual healthcare plan for allergic children at school: lessons from a 2015-2016 school year survey. Pediatr Allergy Immunol. 2017;28(7):655–60.
9. Hogue SL, Muniz R, Herrem C, Silvia S, White MV. Barriers to the administration of epinephrine in schools. J Sch Health. 2018;88(5):396–404.
10. Hogue SL, Goss D, Hollis K, Silvia S, White MV. Training and administration of epinephrine auto-injectors for anaphylaxis treatment in US schools: results from the EpiPen4Schools(®) pilot survey. J Asthma Allergy. 2016;9:109–15.
11. Nowak-Wegrzyn A, Conover-Walker MK, Wood RA. Food-allergic reactions in schools and preschools. Arch Pediatr Adolesc Med. 2001;155(7):790–5.
12. Sicherer SH, Furlong TJ, DeSimone J, Sampson HA. The US Peanut and Tree Nut Allergy Registry: characteristics of reactions in schools and day care. J Pediatr. 2001;138(4):560–5.
13. Redmond M, Kempe E, Strothman K, Wada K, Scherzer R, Stukus DR. Food allergy prevalence and management at an overnight summer camp. Ann Allergy Asthma Immunol. 2016;116(6):518–22.e3.
14. Aktas ON, Kao LM, Hoyt A, Siracusa M, Maloney R, Gupta RS. Development and implementation of an allergic reaction reporting tool for school health personnel: a Pilot Study of Three Chicago Schools. J Sch Nurs. 2018;35:316. https://doi.org/10.1177/1059840518777303.
15. Vale S, Smith J, Said M, Dunne G, Mullins R, Loh R. ASCIA guidelines for prevention of anaphylaxis in schools, pre-schools and childcare: 2012 update: ASCIA anaphylaxis prevention guidelines. J Paediatr Child Health. 2013;49(5):342–5.
16. Grabenhenrich LB, et al. Anaphylaxis in children and adolescents: The European Anaphylaxis Registry. J Allergy Clin Immunol. 2016;137(4):1128–37.e1.
17. Simons FER, et al. World allergy organization anaphylaxis guidelines: 2013 update of the evidence base. Int Arch Allergy Immunol. 2013;162(3):193–204.
18. González-Pérez A, Aponte Z, Vidaurre CF, Rodríguez LAG. Anaphylaxis epidemiology in patients with and patients without asthma: a United Kingdom database review. J Allergy Clin Immunol. 2010;125(5):1098–104.e1.
19. Simons FER, et al. International consensus on (ICON) anaphylaxis. World Allergy Organ J. 2014;7(1):9.
20. Gülen T, Hägglund H, Dahlén B, Nilsson G. High prevalence of anaphylaxis in patients with systemic mastocytosis – a single-centre experience. Clin Exp Allergy J Br Soc Allergy Clin Immunol. 2014;44(1):121–9.
21. Wölbing F, Biedermann T. Anaphylaxis: opportunities of stratified medicine for diagnosis and risk assessment. Allergy. 2013;68(12):1499–508.
22. McWilliam VL, et al. Self-reported adverse food reactions and anaphylaxis in the SchoolNuts study: a population-based study of adolescents. J Allergy Clin Immunol. 2018;141(3):982–90.

23. Motosue MS, Bellolio MF, Van Houten HK, Shah ND, Campbell RL. Increasing emergency department visits for anaphylaxis, 2005–2014. J Allergy Clin Immunol Pract. 2017;5(1):171–5.e3.
24. Mullins RJ, Clark S, Camargo CA. Regional variation in epinephrine autoinjector prescriptions in Australia: more evidence for the vitamin D–anaphylaxis hypothesis. Ann Allergy Asthma Immunol. 2009;103(6):488–95.
25. Poulos LM, Waters A-M, Correll PK, Loblay RH, Marks GB. Trends in hospitalizations for anaphylaxis, angioedema, and urticaria in Australia, 1993–1994 to 2004–2005. J Allergy Clin Immunol. 2007;120(4):878–84.
26. Ribeiro-Vaz I, Marques J, Demoly P, Polónia J, Gomes ER. Drug-induced anaphylaxis: a decade review of reporting to the Portuguese Pharmacovigilance Authority. Eur J Clin Pharmacol. 2013;69(3):673–81.
27. Bilò BM, Bonifazi F. Epidemiology of insect-venom anaphylaxis. Curr Opin Allergy Clin Immunol. 2008;8(4):330–7.
28. De Swert LFA, Bullens D, Raes M, Dermaux A-M. Anaphylaxis in referred pediatric patients: demographic and clinical features, triggers, and therapeutic approach. Eur J Pediatr. 2008;167(11):1251–61.
29. Mehr S, Robinson M, Tang M. Doctor–how do I use my EpiPen? Pediatr Allergy Immunol. 2007;18(5):448–52.
30. Pistiner M, Devore CD, Schoessler S. School food allergy and anaphylaxis management for the pediatrician–extending the medical home with critical collaborations. Pediatr Clin North Am. 2015;62(6):1425–39.
31. Leo HL, Clark NM. Addressing food allergy issues within child care centers. Curr Allergy Asthma Rep. 2012;12(4):304–10.
32. Sampson HA, Mendelson L, Rosen JP. Fatal and near-fatal anaphylactic reactions to food in children and adolescents. N Engl J Med. 1992;327(6):380–4.
33. Devetak I, Devetak SP, Vesel T. Future teachers' attitudes and knowledge regarding the management of the potential students' life-threatening allergic reactions in Slovenian Schools. Zdr Varst. 2018;57(3):124–32.
34. Lanser BJ, Covar R, Bird JA. Food allergy needs assessment, training curriculum, and knowledge assessment for child care. Ann Allergy Asthma Immunol. 2016;116(6):533–7.e4.
35. White MV, et al. EpiPen4Schools pilot survey: occurrence of anaphylaxis, triggers, and epinephrine administration in a U.S. school setting. Allergy Asthma Proc. 2015;36(4):306–12.
36. Dumeier HK, et al. Knowledge of allergies and performance in epinephrine auto-injector use: a controlled intervention in preschool teachers. Eur J Pediatr. 2018;177(4):575–81.
37. Australasian Society of Clinical Immunology and Allergy. "ASCIA e-training for anaphylaxis." Anaphylaxis e-training schools and early childhood education/care, (C) ASCIA 2020. https://etraining.allergy.org.au/.
38. Anaphylaxis Campaign. "Allergy Wise for Schools." Anaphylaxis Campaign supporting people at risk of severe allergies, (C) Anaphylaxis Campaign 2019. https://www.anaphylaxis.org.uk/information-training/allergywise-training/for-schools/.
39. Centers for Disease Control and Prevention. "Managing Food Allergies in Schools The Role os School Teachers and ParaEducators." CDC Healthy Schools. U.S. Department of Health & Human Services, https://www.cdc.gov/healthyschools/foodallergies/pdf/teachers_508_tagged.pdf.
40. Centers for Disease Control and Prevention, Voluntary guidelines for managing food allergies in schools and early care and education programs. Atlanta, GA: US Department of Health and Human; 2013.
41. Watson WT, Woodrow A, Stadnyk AW. Removal of peanut allergen Ara h 1 from common hospital surfaces, toys and books using standard cleaning methods. Allergy Asthma Clin Immunol. 2015;11(1):4.
42. Wainstein BK, Kashef S, Ziegler M, Jelley D, Ziegler JB. Frequency and significance of immediate contact reactions to peanut in peanut-sensitive children. Clin Exp Allergy J Br Soc Allergy Clin Immunol. 2007;37(6):839–45.

43. Johnson RM, Barnes CS. Airborne concentrations of peanut protein. Allergy Asthma Proc. 2013;34(1):59–64.
44. Cherkaoui S, et al. Accidental exposures to peanut in a large cohort of Canadian children with peanut allergy. Clin Transl Allergy. 2015;5:16.
45. Banerjee DK, et al. Peanut-free guidelines reduce school lunch peanut contents. Arch Dis Child. 2007;92(11):980–2.
46. Nguyen-Luu NU, et al. Inadvertent exposures in children with peanut allergy. Pediatr Allergy Immunol. 2012;23(2):133–9.
47. Bartnikas LM, et al. Impact of school peanut-free policies on epinephrine administration. J Allergy Clin Immunol. 2017;140(2):465–73.
48. de Silva IL, Mehr SS, Tey D, Tang MLK. Paediatric anaphylaxis: a 5 year retrospective review. Allergy. 2008;63(8):1071–6.
49. Maloney JM, Chapman MD, Sicherer SH. Peanut allergen exposure through saliva: assessment and interventions to reduce exposure. J Allergy Clin Immunol. 2006;118(3):719–24.
50. Noimark L, et al. The use of adrenaline autoinjectors by children and teenagers. Clin Exp Allergy J Br Soc Allergy Clin Immunol. 2012;42(2):284–92.
51. Sampson MA, Muñoz-Furlong A, Sicherer SH. Risk-taking and coping strategies of adolescents and young adults with food allergy. J Allergy Clin Immunol. 2006;117(6):1440–5.
52. Gupta RS. Anaphylaxis in the young adult population. Am J Med. 2014;127(1 Suppl): S17–24.
53. Dyer AA, O'Keefe A, Kanaley MK, Kao LM, Gupta RS. Leaving the nest: improving food allergy management on college campuses. Ann Allergy Asthma Immunol. 2018;121(1):82–9.e5.
54. Karam M, Scherzer R, Ogbogu PU, Green TD, Greenhawt M. Food allergy prevalence, knowledge, and behavioral trends among college students — a 6-year comparison. J Allergy Clin Immunol Pract. 2017;5(2):504–6.e5.
55. Jevon P, Dimond B. Anaphylaxis: A Practical Guide. Ann Arbor MI: Butterworth-Heinemann Medical; 2004.
56. Feuille E, Lawrence C, Volel C, Sicherer SH, Wang J. Time trends in food allergy diagnoses, epinephrine orders, and epinephrine administrations in New York City schools. J Pediatr. 2017;190:93–9.
57. Le T-M, et al. Low preparedness for food allergy as perceived by school staff: a EuroPrevall survey across Europe. J Allergy Clin Immunol Pract. 2014;2(4):480–2.e1.
58. Moritz S, Schoessler S. Steps to stock: keeping students safe with fully implemented stock epinephrine. NASN Sch Nurse Print. 2018;33(5):268–71.
59. Maughan ED, McCarthy AM, Hein M, Perkhounkova Y, Kelly MW. Medication management in schools: 2015 survey results. J Sch Nurs. 2018;34(6):468–79.
60. Wang J, Bingemann T, Russell AF, Young MC, Sicherer SH. The allergist's role in anaphylaxis and food allergy management in the school and childcare setting. J Allergy Clin Immunol Pract. 2018;6(2):427–35.
61. Sicherer SH, Noone SA, Muñoz-Furlong A. The impact of childhood food allergy on quality of life. Ann Allergy Asthma Immunol. 2001;87(6):461–4.
62. Howe L, Franxman T, Teich E, Greenhawt M. What affects quality of life among caregivers of food-allergic children? Ann Allergy Asthma Immunol. 2014;113(1):69–74.e2.
63. Flokstra-de Blok BMJ, et al. Health-related quality of life of food allergic patients measured with generic and disease-specific questionnaires. Allergy. 2010;65(8):1031–8.
64. Bollinger ME, Dahlquist LM, Mudd K, Sonntag C, Dillinger L, McKenna K. The impact of food allergy on the daily activities of children and their families. Ann Allergy Asthma Immunol. 2006;96(3):415–21.
65. Shah SS, Parker CL, O'Brian Smith E, Davis CM. Disparity in the availability of injectable epinephrine in a large, diverse US school district. J Allergy Clin Immunol Pract. 2014;2(3):288–93.e1.
66. Ford LS, Turner PJ, Campbell DE. Recommendations for the management of food allergies in a preschool/childcare setting and prevention of anaphylaxis. Expert Rev Clin Immunol. 2014;10(7):867–74.

67. Young MC, Muñoz-Furlong A, Sicherer SH. Management of food allergies in schools: a per-spective for allergists. J Allergy Clin Immunol. 2009;124(2):175–82, 182.e1–4; quiz 183–4

68. Langford R, et al. The World Health Organization's Health Promoting Schools framework: a Cochrane systematic review and meta-analysis. BMC Public Health. 2015;15:130.

69. Holt MK, Finkelhor D, Kantor GK. Multiple victimization experiences of urban elementary school students: associations with psychosocial functioning and academic performance. Child Abuse Negl. 2007;31(5):503–15.

70. Mustafa SS, et al. Parent perspectives on school food allergy policy. BMC Pediatr. 2018;18(1):164.

71. Egan M, Sicherer S. Doctor, my child is bullied: food allergy management in schools. Curr Opin Allergy Clin Immunol. 2016;16(3):291–6.

72. Sicherer SH, Mahr T, American Academy of Pediatrics Section on Allergy and Immunology. Management of food allergy in the school setting. Pediatrics. 2010;126(6):1232–9.

73. Ebisawa M, Ito K, Fujisawa T. Japanese guidelines for food allergy 2017. Allergol Int. 2017;66(2):248–64.

74. Anaphylaxis in schools and other childcare settings. AAAAI Board of Directors. American Academy of Allergy, Asthma and Immunology. J Allergy Clin Immunol. 1998;102(2):173–6.

75. Sicherer SH, Simons FER, SECTION ON ALLERGY AND IMMUNOLOGY. Epinephrine for first-aid management of anaphylaxis. Pediatrics. 2017;139(3):e20164006.

76. Wang J, Sicherer SH, SECTION ON ALLERGY AND IMMUNOLOGY. Guidance on com-pleting a written allergy and anaphylaxis emergency plan. Pediatrics. 2017;139(3):e20164005.

77. Vale S, Smith J, Said M, Mullins RJ, Loh R. ASCIA guidelines for prevention of anaphylaxis in schools, pre-schools and childcare: 2015 update. J Paediatr Child Health. 2015;51(10):949–54.

78. Muraro A, et al. EAACI food allergy and anaphylaxis guidelines: managing patients with food allergy in the community. Allergy. 2014;69(8):1046–57.

Advocacy for Anaphylaxis

9

Tonya Winders and Stanley Fineman

Rationale for Advocacy

Never doubt that a small group of thoughtful committed citizens can change the world; indeed, it's the only thing that ever has.– Margaret Mead

Advocacy is defined as "a coordinated combination of problem identification, solution creation, strategy development, and actions taken to make positive change." Two types of advocacy are most relevant for the physician community to understand throughout this chapter.

Health Advocacy

- Enhancing community health and policy initiatives that focus on the availability, safety, and quality of care

Legislative Advocacy

- Reliance on legislative processes (state or federal) as a strategy to create change

  Advocacy can take place at any level—local, state, federal, and international. Throughout this chapter, we will explore general advocacy approaches for each and highlight success stories across North America.

T. Winders
Allergy & Asthma Network, Global Allergy & Airways Patient Platform, Vienna, VA, USA
e-mail: twinders@allergyasthmanetwork.org

S. Fineman (✉)
Emory University School of Medicine, Atlanta Allergy & Asthma, Vienna, VA, USA
e-mail: SFineman@atlantaallergy.com

© Springer Nature Switzerland AG 2020
A. K. Ellis (ed.), *Anaphylaxis*, https://doi.org/10.1007/978-3-030-43205-8_9

   Physicians are important advocates at the local level. As an advocate for the patient, "the concerns and best interests of the patient are at the core of all decisions and interactions" [1]. Physicians should listen to their patients, respect their autonomy and beliefs, and allow patients to be fully involved in their healthcare decisions. Making decisions for patients or withholding key medical information is not being an advocate for their patient, and it does not allow the patient to be an advocate for themselves. It is imperative to engage in a shared decision-making process to marry the best scientific evidence with an individual patient's preferences, values, and beliefs [2]. The American College of Asthma, Allergy & Immunology partnered with Allergy & Asthma Network to develop shared decision aids for the severe asthma, allergen immunotherapy, and atopic dermatitis [3].

   Key components of a local physician advocate include the following [1]:

- Inform the patient and promote informed consent.
- Empower the patient and protect autonomy.
- Protect the rights and interests of the patients where they cannot protect their own.
- Ensure patients have fare access to available resources.
- Support the patient no matter what the potential cost.
- Represent the views/desires of the patient and not just his/her needs.

   Advocating for the patient is not pushing him/her toward one outcome, right or wrong; it is giving him/her all the information and resources to give her the opportunity to make the best decision for the patient and their family.

   At the levels, physicians have the unique opportunity to share our expertise, advocate for our patients and our field, and educate our lawmakers. It is important to share your voice, contact your representative, and/or lobby on legislation that affects our field, our patients, and the care we provide. Every day there are rules, regulations, laws, and programs that are being implemented and/or changed by government entities that affect the practice of not only Allergy & Clinical Immunology but all fields of medicine. Through advocacy, a physician's rights and needs are expressed and represented. By advocating for what is and/or is not an appropriate course of action, a physician serves as the expert and provides insight that would otherwise not be considered.

   Advocacy for anaphylaxis is needed. It is now estimated that 15 million Americans are living with a life-threatening food allergy. Many more are at risk of anaphylaxis due to medications, latex, and insect allergic reactions. Given the continued rise in prevalence and greater awareness of morbidity and mortality due to anaphylaxis, now is the time to let your voice be heard as a physician advocate.

General Advocacy Approaches

Advocacy is not lobbying. Lobbying refers specifically to advocacy efforts that attempt to influence legislation. This distinction is helpful to keep in mind because it means that laws limiting the lobbying done by nonprofit organizations do not govern other advocacy activities. When nonprofit organizations advocate on their own behalf, they seek to affect some aspect of society, whether they appeal to individuals about their behavior, employers about their rules, or the government about its laws.

Before we discuss the important of state and federal advocacy in detail, it is important to review how bills become laws to better understand how physicians can advocate for legislation that affects our field and our patients.

Local and state government officials are elected by their city, county/parish, or district. Federal government structure is comprised of 435 members in the US House of Representatives who serve 2-year terms with no limit to the number of terms one can serve. The US Senate is comprised of 100 members who serve 6-year terms. Each year one-third of the Senate is up for re-election. Once again there is no limit to the number of terms one can serve.

Local

Physicians should be knowledgeable and stay informed regarding local advocacy opportunities. Many things can be done daily to advance anaphylaxis awareness and preparedness. For example, in your own practice, you can encourage the use of anaphylaxis action plans or host educational events for schools, daycares, camps, etc. You can be a resource for local media or utilize your own social media to amplify guideline-based approaches to care.

Moreover, physicians should attend town hall meetings or invite legislators to work with you for a tour or shadowing to better understand the challenges in health-care today. It is important to develop relationships with your legislator's local staff, attend fundraisers, and support candidates who align with your views. Calls, emails, and letters to legislators are often called "grassroots advocacy" and are still very effective ways to get your point across.

Local examples of advocacy for those at risk of anaphylaxis abound. One of the most well-recognized programs is the Anaphylaxis Community Experts (ACE) program which has been organized by Allergy & Asthma Network and run successfully since 2012. The ACE program consists of over 300 physician-led teams throughout the United States and has over 1000 volunteers including physicians, school nurses, patients, parents, etc. These teams have directly trained over one million people in recognizing the signs, symptoms, causes, and treatment for ana-phylaxis. Moreover, the ACE volunteers often conduct media interviews and attend local health fairs or community events to heighten awareness of anaphy-laxis [4].

Beyond Your Local Community

To be a more effective medical advocate, it is critical to understand how bills become laws to better understand how physicians can advocate for legislation that affects our field and our patients. Any senator or representative can develop a legislative proposal. Once introduced, it becomes a bill and is assigned a unique number. House bills begin with H.R. and Senate bills begin with S. Bill sponsors can then recruit other members to support and cosponsor legislation.

Committee chairs have several options when considering a bill. They can choose to hold a hearing on a bill, or they can schedule a "markup" of a bill where committee members can offer amendments, change the bill, and send the bill to the full House or Senate for floor vote. Finally, they can also choose to take no action on a bill. On occasion the house speaker or senate majority leader may choose to bypass committees and bring legislation directly to floor for a vote.

Passage of most bills in the House requires a simple majority. The House has rules including the number of amendments that can be offered on the floor and a time limit on how long a bill can be debated.

On the other hand, the Senate has very few rules regarding consideration of a bill. First, any senator can amend, slow down, or stop a bill at any time. A senator stands on Senate floor and speaks without resting for the entire time if he or she wants to delay the action on a bill. This is called filibustering. Only a cloture vote, requiring 60 votes, can end a filibuster. If 60 votes are not obtained, the bill will be pulled from the floor with no further action.

When the House and Senate pass different versions of the same bill, it must be conferenced. This is a process for reconciling two bills into a common text that can be voted on again by both bodies. It should be noted that the House and Senate leaders of both parties appoint members to the conference committee. Only when passed in identical form by both chambers does a bill go to the president for signature. The president then has 10 days except Sundays to sign a bill into law or to veto the bill.

When a bill is vetoed, it is sent back to the Congress and can become a law if it wins a two-thirds approval from the House and Senate.

State

Advocacy at the state level can include visits to your state's legislature in Capitol Hill and participating in campaign efforts by making introductions, donating, and voting for candidates who prioritize healthcare issues.

Advocacy for anaphylaxis at the state level is where significant progress has occurred in the last 5 to 10 years. For example, all patient advocacy organizations and the physician community joined forces to advance students' ability to self-carry epinephrine and access to stock epinephrine in schools [5]. Today, all 50 states have a law which allows students to self-carry their emergency medication with them at school rather than forcing them to store it in a central location such as the office or with the school nurse. Furthermore, 49 states now have legislation in place which allows the school to stock epinephrine to use in the event of an emergency even in the absence of a prescription for that individual. These measures have ensured that countless lives were saved because in the case of anaphylaxis, minutes matter [6]. Quick and easy access to emergency medication is lifesaving.

Without the aid of physicians advocating for proper care of anaphylaxis by providing expert testimony, writing letters, and making visits and calls to their state houses, this would not have occurred.

Federal

In the federal government, several members hold influential roles including the speaker of the house and senate majority leader, US house majority leader, US house minority leader, majority whip, minority whip, caucus chair, and the conference chair. On the Senate side, additional leadership roles include president (who is the US vice-president), president pro tempore, majority leader, minority leader, majority whip, and the minority whip.

Below is the chart of the committees in the House and Senate:

House Committees
1. Energy and Commerce
2. Ways and Means
3. Budget
4. House Appropriations
5. House Science
6. Government Reform
7. Judiciary
8. Small Business

Senate Committees
1. Finance
2. Health, Education, Labor and Pensions (HELP)
3. Budget
4. Appropriations Committees

In the House of Representatives, health legislation typically goes through Energy and Commerce and/or Ways and Means. Energy and Commerce committee has a health subcommittee and has jurisdiction over Medicare Part B which includes physician payment, Medicaid, food and drug safety, and public health. The Ways and Means Committee has jurisdiction over taxes. It also has a health subcommittee which oversees Medicare Part A (hospitals) and Part B (physician payment). The Budget Committee directs government spending to particular programs.

In the Senate, health legislation typically goes to the Senate Finance Committee or the Health, Education, Labor and Pensions Committee. The Senate Finance Committee has jurisdiction over Medicare, Medicaid, and the State Children's Health Insurance Program (SCHIP) and jurisdiction over health programs financed by specific tax or trust funds. The HELP Committee has jurisdiction over public health and health insurance and over most of the agencies, institutes, and programs of the DHHS, including FDA, CDC, and NIH. Lastly, the Budget and Appropriations Committees are also important to healthcare issues due to appropriations spending.

Timing is always important, and anaphylaxis advocacy in the Congress is no exception. The Congress convenes every odd year for a 2-year period (e.g. 116th Congress runs from Jan. 2018–Dec. 2019 with first and second sessions). Legislation introduced during the first session can be carried over to second session; however, the slate is wiped clean at the end of the second session, and unfinished bills must be reintroduced. Majority party leader in each house also has control over that chamber's schedule.

When it comes to success stories in federal advocacy specific to anaphylaxis, many examples come to mind. First, in 2004, the federal government passed the Asthmatic Schoolchildren's Treatment and Health Management Act (ASTHMA) [5]. This created an incentive for states to pass a law allowing students to self-carry emergency medicines for allergies and asthma on their person at school. Surveys, posters, briefings, speeches, and media efforts resulted in President Bush signing the law into effect and set the stage for all 50 states to do the same over the next 10 years.

In 2013, the School Access to Emergency Epinephrine Act passage sparked a nationwide movement to allow or require schools to stock emergency supplies of epinephrine to treat anaphylaxis [6]. In 2018, 49 states have followed suit, and only Hawaii remains until all students have the ability to benefit from this lifesaving policy.

Physician advocates have also spoken out at the Food and Drug Administration at advisory committee meetings for new drug applications or over-the-counter application proceedings. Currently, the patient advocacy community is working to get sesame labeling enacted by the FDA. Each year, physicians participate in the annual Allergy & Asthma Day on Capitol Hill to highlight challenges facing the medical community and patients. Some of these topics have advocated for access to epinephrine via the drug price transparency and nonmedical switching policy debates. It is always beneficial to have an expert opinion to reinforce the need for anaphylaxis awareness and preparedness given the rise of life-threatening allergies in North America.

International

There are numerous opportunities for physicians to get involved in advocacy for anaphylaxis on international issues. This most often takes place by letter writing campaigns to either the US national leaders or international leaders. If you have an international policy concern, it is always a good idea to notify your representative or the executive branch through email and phone calls or schedule an in-person visit. Sign-on petitions have also been effective to change policy. Finally, volunteering to work with international organizations will allow firsthand experience in advocating. The World Allergy Organization is a valuable resource for identifying how to get involved on a global level.

One North American success story is the collaboration between Food Allergy Canada and Allergy & Asthma Network in the United States to co-develop and disseminate *Living Confidently with Food Allergy* by Dr. Michael Pistiner and Dr. Jennifer LeBovidge from Boston, Massachusetts [7]. Over 10,000 booklets were shared with patients and families from 2014 to 2016. Another success is in the area of national guideline documents, physicians advocated in both Canada and the United States to ensure national guidelines on the diagnosis and treatment of anaphylaxis were adopted and implemented.

Food Allergy Research & Education (FARE) also is leading a current effort to share research findings and raise awareness globally by working with Global Allergy Asthma Patient Platform (GAAPP) and international food allergy patient organizations such as Anaphylaxis Canada, Food Allergy Italia, Allergy UK, and others. This effort is critical to not only understanding the continued rise in prevalence and increase in burden globally but also gaining resources globally to address the unmet needs.

Summary

By understanding the principals of advocacy, including health advocacy for patients as well as legislative advocacy that helps develop policies, physicians can have a positive impact in the care of patients with anaphylaxis.

Tools and Resources for Anaphylaxis Advocates
Websites

Allergy & Asthma Network	www.AllergyAsthmaNetwork.org
AllergyHome	www.AllergyHome.org
American Academy of Allergy, Asthma & Immunology	www.AAAAI.org
American College of Allergy, Asthma & Immunology	www.ACAAI.org
Asthma and Allergy Foundation of America	www.AAFA.org
Centers for Disease Control and Prevention	www.cdc.gov/healthyschools/foodallergies
Food Allergy & Anaphylaxis Connection Team	www.foodalleergyawareness.org
Food Allergy Canada	www.FoodAllergyCanada.ca
Food Allergy Research & Education	www.FoodAllergy.org
Guidelines for the Diagnosis and Management of Food Allergy in the United States	www.niaid.nih.gov/topics/foodallergy
National Association of School Nurses	www.nasn.org/toolsresources/foodallergyandanaphylaxis

Publications and Posters

AAFA Online Community and Newly Diagnosed Education	www.kidswithfoodallergies.org
Allergy & Anaphylaxis: A Practical Guide for Schools and Families	www.members.allergyasthmanetwork.org/store
Allergy-Safe Dining: A Guide for the Food Service Industry	www.members.allergyasthmanetwork.org/store

Anaphylaxis At A Glance Poster	www.members.allergyasthmanetwork.org/store
FAACT School Programs and Posters	www.foodallergyawareness.org/education/education-resource-center/
Food Allergy 101, Emergency Care Plan and Advocacy Toolbox	www.foodallergy.org/education-awareness/
Information sheets, webinars, and online support	www.foodallergycanada.ca/resources/print-materials/
Living Confidently with Food Allergy	www.foodallergycanada.ca/resources/newly-diagnosed-handbook/
Living with Latex Allergy	www.members.allergyasthmanetwork.org/store
Understanding Anaphylaxis	www.members.allergyasthmanetwork.org/store

References

1. Schwartz L. Is there an advocate in the house? The role of health care professionals in patient advocacy. J Med Ethics. 2002;28:37–40.
2. https://www.healthit.gov/sites/default/files/nlc_shared_decision_making_fact_sheet.pdf.
3. http://severeasthmatreatments.chestnet.org.
4. http://www.allergyasthmanetwork.org/outreach/anaphylaxis-community-experts-aces/.
5. http://www.allergyasthmanetwork.org/advocacy/current-issues/medications-school/.
6. http://www.allergyasthmanetwork.org/advocacy/current-issues/stock-epinephrine/.
7. www.foodallergycanada.ca/resources/newly-diagnosed-handbook/.

Resources for Anaphylaxis

10

Anne K. Ellis

In this brief section, we have highlighted key review articles that have been heavily cited throughout the text book as well as provided a list of online resources that should prove helpful to practitioners and patients alike.

Websites

AAAAI: American Academy of Allergy, Asthma & Immunology – A membership organization of more than 7000 allergists/immunologists and patient's trusted resource for allergies, asthma, and immune deficiency disorders. https://aaaai.org

ACAAI: American College of Allergy, Asthma & Immunology – The ACAAI is a professional medical organization of more than 6000 allergists/immunologists and allied health professionals. Members live and practice throughout the United States and internationally. The College fosters a culture of collaboration and congeniality in which its members work together, and with others, toward the common goals of patient care, education, advocacy, and research. ACAAI allergists are board-certified physicians trained to diagnose allergies and asthma, administer immunotherapy, and provide patients with the best treatment outcomes. https://acaai.org/

AAFA: The Asthma and Allergy Foundation of America, a not-for-profit organization founded in 1953, is the leading patient organization for people with asthma and allergies and the oldest asthma and allergy patient group in the world. https://www.aafa.org/

AllergyHome: At AllergyHome, we are part of a community striving to keep our kids with food allergies strong, safe, and healthy. We know the challenges that come with managing pediatric food allergies and life-threatening anaphylaxis. Sharing

A. K. Ellis (✉)
Queen's University, Kingston, ON, Canada
e-mail: Anne.Ellis@kingstonhsc.ca

© Springer Nature Switzerland AG 2020
A. K. Ellis (ed.), *Anaphylaxis*, https://doi.org/10.1007/978-3-030-43205-8_10

expert-guided knowledge, experiences, and tools, you can be assured that AllergyHome's resources can assist you in protecting and empowering your children and community living with food allergies. https://Allergyhome.org/

CSACI: The Canadian Society of Allergy and Clinical Immunology is one of the oldest specialty societies in Canada. It was founded in 1945 as the Canadian Society for the Study of Allergy and changed its name in 1954 to the Canadian Academy of Allergy. In 1967, it adopted the present name, The Canadian Society of Allergy and Clinical Immunology (CSACI).

The goals of the society are to:

- Improve the standards of teaching and practice of allergy and clinical immunology. Foster cooperation between those engaged in the study and practice of allergy and clinical immunology.
- Encourage research in the field of allergy and clinical immunology.
- Promote harmony and understanding between physicians engaged in the practice of allergy and clinical immunology and others of the medical profession. https://csaci.ca

FARE: Food Allergy Research and Education – FARE's mission is to improve the quality of life and the health of individuals with food allergies and to provide them hope through the promise of new treatments. https://foodallergy.org

Food Allergy Canada: Food Allergy Canada is a nonprofit organization dedicated to helping Canadians with food allergies live with confidence. https://foodallergy-canada.ca/

Suggested Reading

1. Lieberman P, Nicklas RA, Randolph C, Oppenheimer J, et al. Anaphylaxis–a practice parameter update 2015. Ann Allergy Asthma Immunol. 2015;115(5):341–84.
2. Fischer D, Vander Leek TK, Ellis AK, Kim H. Anaphylaxis. Allergy Asthma Clin Immunol. 2018;14(Suppl 2):54.
3. Simons FE, Ardusso LR, Dimov V, et al. World Allergy Organization Anaphylaxis Guidelines: 2013 update of the evidence base. Int Arch Allergy Immunol. 2013;162(3):193–204.
4. Sicherer SH, Simons FER. Epinephrine for first-aid management of anaphylaxis. Pediatrics. 2017;139(3):e20164006.
5. Greenhawt M, Gupta RS, Meadows JA, et al. Guiding principles for the recognition, diagnosis, and management of infants with anaphylaxis: an Expert Panel Consensus. J Allergy Clin Immunol Pract. 2019;7(4):1148–56.e5.
6. Lieberman P, Simons FE. Anaphylaxis and cardiovascular disease: therapeutic dilemmas. Clin Exp Allergy. 2015;45(8):1288–95.
7. Alqurashi W, Ellis AK. Do corticosteroids prevent biphasic anaphylaxis? J Allergy Clin Immunol Pract. 2017;5(5):1194–205.
8. Pourmand A, Robinson C, Syed W, Mazer-Amirshahi M. Biphasic anaphylaxis: a review of the literature and implications for emergency management. Am J Emerg Med. 2018;36(8):1480–5.
9. Lee S, Bellolio MF, Hess EP, et al. Time of onset and predictors of biphasic anaphylactic reactions: a systematic review and meta-analysis. J Allergy Clin Immunol Pract. 2015;3(3):408–16.e1–2.

10. Muñoz-Cano R, Pascal M, Araujo G, et al. Mechanisms, cofactors, and augmenting factors involved in anaphylaxis. Front Immunol. 2017;8:1193.
11. Ansley L, Bonini M, Delgado L, et al. Pathophysiological mechanisms of exercise-induced anaphylaxis: an EAACI position statement. Allergy. 2015;70(10):1212–21.
12. Greenberger PA, Lieberman P. Idiopathic anaphylaxis. J Allergy Clin Immunol Pract. 2014;2(3):243–50.
13. Grabenhenrich LB, Dölle S, Moneret-Vautrin A, et al. Anaphylaxis in children and adolescents: The European Anaphylaxis Registry. J Allergy Clin Immunol. 2016;137(4):1128–37.e1.
14. Cohen N, Capua T, Pivko D, et al. Trends in the diagnosis and management of anaphylaxis in a tertiary care pediatric emergency department. Ann Allergy Asthma Immunol. 2018;121(3):348–52.
15. Waserman S, Avilla E, Ben-Shoshan M, et al. Epinephrine autoinjectors: new data, new problems. J Allergy Clin Immunol Pract. 2017;5(5):1180–91.
16. Hochstadter E, Clarke A, De Schryver S, et al. Increasing visits for anaphylaxis and the benefits of early epinephrine administration: a 4-year study at a pediatric emergency department in Montreal, Canada. J Allergy Clin Immunol. 2016;137(6):1888–90.e4.
17. Mawhirt SL, Fonacier L, Aquino M. Utilization of high-fidelity simulation for medical student and resident education of allergic-immunologic emergencies. Ann Allergy Asthma Immunol. 2019;122(5):513–21.
18. Scherber RM, Borate U. How we diagnose and treat systemic mastocytosis in adults. Br J Haematol. 2018;180(1):11–23.
19. Abid A, Malone MA, Curci K. Mastocytosis. Prim Care. 2016;43(3):505–18.

Index

© Springer Nature Switzerland AG 2020
A. K. Ellis (ed.), *Anaphylaxis*, https://doi.org/10.1007/978-3-030-43205-8

The manufacturer's authorised representative in the EU is Springer Nature Customer Service Centre GmbH, Europaplatz 3, 69115 Heidelberg, Germany. If you have any concerns regarding our products, please contact ProductSafety@springernature.com

Printed and bound by CPI Group (UK) Ltd, Croydon, CR0 4YY

29/04/2026

02099451-0015